PROJECT 2000: REFLECTION AND CELEBRATION

Project 2000: reflection and celebration

Edited by
Brian Dolan, RMN, RGN, CHSM

Foreword by
Betty Kershaw, MSc, SRN, RCNT, RNT, DANS, OND

Scutari Press
London

© Scutari Press 1993

Published by Scutari Press, a division of Scutari Projects Ltd. the publishing company of the Royal College of Nursing, London

First published 1993

British Library Cataloguing in Publication Data
Dolan, Brian
    Project 2000: Reflection and Celebration
    I. Title
    610.73

    ISBN 1–871364–81–7

Typeset by J&L Composition Ltd, Filey, North Yorkshire
Printed by Loader Jackson, Bedfordshire

DEDICATION

To my mother: For all the joy and laughter she brought into the lives of those of us who knew her and whom I was privileged to nurse in her final illness.

To my father: For showing dignity, strength and wisdom when there was, and still is, pain at the loss of a wife and friend of 43 years. A father any son would be proud to have.

Contents

Contributors   viii

Foreword — Betty Kershaw   ix

Introduction   1

Chapter 1. **Reflection and Celebration** Brian Dolan   3

Chapter 2. **Power, Politics and Peril** John Naish   17

Chapter 3. **All Change — Project 2000's Greatest Challenge?**
            Jill E Robinson   31

Chapter 4. **The Challenge of Higher Education**
            Jan Charlwood   47

Chapter 5. **Empowerment: Taking Chances, Making
            Changes** Charlotte Allen   57

Chapter 6. **Gender and Change** Brian Dolan   75

Chapter 7. **A Reflection on Issues for Practice**
            Pippa Gough, Sian Maslin-Prothero and
            Abigail Masterson   89

Chapter 8. **Into the Community** June Clark   107

Chapter 9. **The Changing Face of Nursing — 2000 and
            Beyond** Jean Thomas and Brian Dolan   121

Appendix I   131

Appendix II   135

Appendix III   137

Index   139

Contributors

Charlotte Allen BA, MA
Project 2000 student, Leeds College of Health

Jan Charlwood BSc(Hons), RGN
Lecturer in Nursing, Southampton College of Nursing

June Clark PhD, BA(Hons), CHSM, RN, FRCN
Professor of Nursing and Health Care Studies, Middlesex University

Pippa Gough MPS, RGN, RM, HV, PGCEA
Project Worker, King's Fund Centre

Sian Maslin-Prothero RGN, RM, DipN(Lond)
Nurse Teacher, Avon College of Health

Abigail Masterson BSc, RGN, PGCEA
Lecturer, Institute of Advanced Nursing Education, Royal College of Nursing

John Naish BA(Hons)
Viewpoint Editor, *Nursing Standard*
Editor, *Tradimus*, the RCN Association of Nursing Students Journal

Jill E Robinson BSc(Hons), CertEd, RMN
Senior Research Associate, the Suffolk and Great Yarmouth College of Nursing and Midwifery

Jean Thomas DipN(Lond), RCNT, ONC, RGN
Assistant Director, Nursing Policy and Practice, Royal College of Nursing

Brian Dolan RMN, RGN, CHSM
Clinical Consultant, *Nursing Standard*, formerly Student Association Officer, Royal College of Nursing

Foreword

Project 2000 is all about change: change in education, change in practice, change (one hopes) in the way care is delivered. It was planned as a precursor to support the many recent Government initiatives, including 'Care in the Community', The Patient's Charter, with its emphasis on the named nurse, and 'The Health of the Nation'. The curriculum for the courses supports an individual, community-based, health promotional approach to the practice of nursing, and emphasises personal/professional responsibility and accountability. It aims to produce assertive nurses, with skills in counselling and advocacy, who are able to take through to registration their expertise in all these complex areas of care and who are motivated (and capable) self-directed learners, able to develop their competence on their own iniative.

All this is indeed change, and change of a very fundamental kind in that it moves the perspective of nursing through almost one hundred and eighty degrees from a hospital-based medically modelled approach to treatment and care. Of course, not all this happened at once, but for those who trained in the 1960's and 1970's it has happened in our professional lifetime.

Change produces anxiety, stress and of course, excitement. We all react to it in different ways – after all one man's meat is another man's poison – and all of us view it from different perspectives, seeing different issues of importance. This book aims to explore these many and varied issues from the viewpoint of those involved in and with them. It includes contributions from students, teachers, managers and practitioners, all bringing to the text a unique and personal opinion. Fundamental to their work is the delivery of care at the patient/client level. The chapters aim to assist the reader to reflect (definitely the 'in' word of the 1990's) on the success and indeed the shortcomings of the programme to date and to ponder on improvements which could usefully be made. From such critical analysis the book aims to show where we should go next, recognising that the profession needs both courage and belief in itself if it is to use the past to map out the future.

Project 2000 is seen as much more than 'just another course'. It is a revolution, celebrating the growth of our profession in its movement to meet the health care needs of this decade and beyond.

In order to edit such a book, Brian Dolan has collected together an impressive list of contributors. June Clark reflects on, reacts to and debates the enormous field of community care; all her comments are research-based and grounded in clinical practice. This reflection follows an exploration of the broader interests of practice-based education. Interestingly, the book is really in three sections, the first three chapters addressing the political and cultural change that has taken, and is indeed taking place, reflecting on the whole issue of constant and at times rushed and seemingly unplanned change.

The second three chapters are perhaps the most interesting in that they 'tease out' some of the professional issues which impact with this massive programme of change. Charlotte Allen, a Project 2000 student, challenges some of the 'Ivory Towers' professionals have, especially the 'teacher knows best' and 'do as Sister tells you' approach to education. It is refreshing to explore the value she places on students' own knowledge and what they bring to the profession. She must be reassured that some new thoughts do exist in the fields of management, education and practice as she reads the contributions of her fellow authors. The final chapter aims to stimulate debate, raising questions not answers, and challenging teachers to move forward.

This is a challenging book, not least in that it doesn't always make a comfortable read!

Have you the courage to take up the challenge?

Betty Kershaw
1993

Introduction

If Project 2000 is the answer, what on earth was the question? Well you may ask, for until now the answer has hardly been forthcoming.

In many ways this book was born out of a growing realisation that Project 2000, the biggest change to nurse education, is poorly understood and all too often maligned. Sometimes by those who ought to know better, but more often by those who simply do not, because there was no one to answer the questions.

This book has two purposes; first, to reflect on where we have been. It looks around to show us where we are and it looks forward to show us where we could go — if we have the courage and faith to do so. Second, it celebrates our growing confidence in ourselves as a profession, in the way Project 2000 is a celebration of faith in our future. Project 2000 is more than an educational foundation, it is a platform from which nursing can launch itself to the self-confidence, self-belief and self-awareness that becomes a profession.

The contributors to this book have been approached because they all bring unique perspectives of Project 2000. By drawing together experts from practice, education, research and management, as well as those with political insights into the world of nursing, you are offered a view of a profession that is slowly, but very surely, coming to believe in itself as a force for real change.

If you are expecting to read a sanitised version of nursing or Project 2000, you will (hopefully) be disappointed. Life, just like nursing, is simply not like that and to pretend, or ask the contributors to do otherwise, would be less than honest. Instead, you will be offered a view that is realistic, frank, occasionally controversial, but most of all affirming in its belief in Project 2000 as a catalyst for change.

Although more serendipitous than intentional, the nine chapters of *Project 2000 — Reflection and Celebration* fall neatly into three sections. The first three chapters, in one form or another, examine some of the changes that were, or are, necessary to ensure Project 2000 came to fruition. From its pre-history and political challenges to the opportunities it offers to those who wish to take them, these preliminary chapters highlight how much control the nursing profession has over its own destiny if it can only believe in itself.

The second section teases out some of the professional issues that will inevitably have a significant impact on the success of both Project 2000 and the profession at large, that is education, empowerment and gender. If, for instance, Project 2000 is about education and empowerment, then Charlotte Allen's contribution underlines some of the changes that have already occurred. She has not written because she is a Project 2000 student, for that would be tokenism of the worst kind. Instead, her contribution is included because, like the other chapters, it is original, articulate and passionate about nurses and nursing. If Project 2000 presents a change in the way we educate students, then asking the consumers of that education for their view starts to get us away from the hierarchy bound 'qualified nurses know what is best for students' syndrome. It also erodes the arrogant assumption that students come into the profession as empty vessels waiting to be filled with nursing knowledge, with little to contribute to their own or their profession's advancement.

The final three chapters look at some of the practice issues, present and future, hospital and community based, that face the Project 2000 nurse now and later. The final chapter, however, does not pretend to offer a comprehensive view of the future — only some of those elements the authors felt would stimulate further debate. Looking to the future is becoming a cottage industry in some areas, but we were mindful of Rogers' (1983) exhortation 'to glimpse a becoming, to see with that "third eye" . . . to speculate upon a dream and to watch that dream unfold . . . to create a new reality.'

Project 2000 offers us the opportunity to create that new reality. This book will help us reflect upon where we are going. Most of all, it will let us celebrate what Project 2000 can offer.

REFERENCE

Rogers M E (1983) Beyond the Horizon. In *The Nursing Profession: A Time to Speak* (ed N L Chaska). New York: McGraw Hill.

CHAPTER 1

Reflection and Celebration

Brian Dolan

'The status quo is not an option.' (UKCC 1986)

Project 2000 is an educational programme developed by and for nurses (Mason, 1991). Its purpose is to prepare practitioners who are flexible, autonomous and critically aware of the increasingly complex health care needs of society in the 1990's and beyond.

This chapter will place Project 2000 in a historical context to show how the nursing profession, having decided on its educational destiny, was able to control it. It will highlight the challenges the first Project 2000 students have faced and will explore and debunk some of the myths and misconceptions surrounding the course. In conclusion, drawing on research from nursing graduate career trajectories, it will be suggested that the career path of Project 2000 practitioners will be a hybrid of both the graduate and conventionally trained nurse.

THE HISTORICAL CONTEXT

The concept of Project 2000 could hardly be described as revolutionary. Its seeds were sown some 50 years ago when the Horder Report (RCN 1943) proposed that the education of nurses should be separated from the needs of the nursing service and that the student nurse be recognised as a student of nursing. However, these seeds of change fell on stony ground and one can only speculate what might have been had this call been heeded half a century ago.

Why the distinction between student nurse and student of nursing? In fact it was, and remains, a critical issue. Nurse training was largely unchanged since Florence Nightingale had set up the first nursing school at St Thomas' Hospital back in the 1860's (Gratian and Holland 1959). It was based on an apprenticeship model of on-the-job training with the student's own educational needs always subordinate to the needs of the service. The difference between studentship and apprenticeship is highlighted in Figure 1.1.

	Studentship	Apprenticeship
Rationale	Command of disciplines	Learn routines
Benefits	To student	To service
Purpose	Understanding	Getting job done
Learning	Intellectual	Play a role
Content	Selective	Complete
Thinking	Conceptual	Tasks
Competence	Transferable skills	Limited repertoire of behavioural skills
Student responsibility	High	Low
Student attitude	Questioning	Passive
Mistakes	Inevitable	Sign of failure

Figure 1.1 The difference between studentship and apprenticeship

As can be seen from Figure 1.1, the difference was not just an exercise in semantics but would require a paradigmatic shift in the way nursing students were viewed. A few years later, the Wood Report on Recruitment and Training of Nurses (Ministry of Health 1947) was more explicit and called for students to have full student status and be supernumerary during practical training. But, as Naish points out in Chapter 2, not only was this report also unheeded, it was actively resisted by the nursing profession, most notably by the General Nursing Council (GNC) and the Royal College of Nursing (RCN), whose ruling councils were dominated by matrons who did not wish to see either their powerbases eroded or the end to what was *de facto* a cheap source of labour for them.

Later still, the Platt Report on Nurse Education (RCN 1964) unambiguously stated that:

'The reconstruction of the existing system (of nurse education) is essential.' (p. 1)

It argued:

'This country has long enjoyed a nursing service at a very low cost because of the use made of student nurses in providing the service. The system can no longer be justified; it is contrary to the best interests of patients and students within a highly developed health service.' (pp. 36–37)

While the RCN leadership was now supportive, the GNC, however, remained unmoved, responding:

'A very great number of those who enter nursing do so with a stronger desire to be a nurse than to be a student, and that if too great an emphasis is placed on the student status of the nurse in training this may in fact act as a deterrent to recruitment.' (*Nursing Times* 1965a, p. 1328)

Students themselves whose own voices were mute, if not muzzled, during these years of lofty debate about their future were also entering the fray. As if to underline the chasm between the GNC's perceived desires of students and the students' own needs, members of the Student Nurses Association (later to become the RCN's Association of Nursing Students), wrote in the *Nursing Times* (1965b):

'There can be no progress in a profession that continues to disregard basic orthodox educational principles in the training of its members.' (p. 1347)

Ironically, this letter appeared only the week before the GNC made its pronouncement that nursing students did not want to be students at all!

Despite the debate it generated, the Platt Report (RCN 1964) was left on the shelf to gather dust. Over the next two decades other reports (Committee on Nursing 1972; Royal Commission in the National Health Service 1979; Committee of Enquiry into Mental Handicap Nursing 1979) referred to, or looked specifically at, nurse education without, it seems, making any significant impact on nursing or government policy. (See Appendix I.) However, as

Mason (1991) notes, dramatic social, technological and medical changes through the latter part of this century necessitated a major rethink in the way nurses were educated. That rethink was to become Project 2000.

A TIME FOR CHANGE

By the 1980's three critical factors made the need for educational reform essential:

1. Demographic changes: that nursing has traditionally relied on large numbers of 18-year-olds with five or more GCSEs, or their equivalent, is hardly surprising. Yet from the mid-1950's the birth rate rose, then fell again steeply by some 35 per cent between 1964 and 1976 (Beardshaw 1992). Relying on its traditional pool of recruits meant that by 1995, 50 per cent of all female school leavers with five GCSEs would need to enter nursing to maintain, much less increase, present staffing levels (O'Connor 1987). Unsurprisingly, a number of writers have doubted that this is possible (Bosanquet 1985; Pearce 1988).
2. Prevention is better than cure: both the government and nursing recognised the need for a shift in emphasis away from the acute hospital setting towards the community provision of health care. The value of ill-health prevention as opposed to ill-health treatment was being increasingly appreciated (UKCC 1987b).
3. Value for money: there was a growing realisation that irrespective of the hue of the political party in power, there was, and would continue to be, a sustained emphasis on cost-effectiveness and value for money (UKCC 1987b).

The RCN, which had been fully committed to the reform of nurse education for some years, in 1984 set up the Judge Commission which reported a year later (Commission on Nurse Education 1985). It was unequivocal in its demands — students should have supernumerary status; there should be one level of nurse; nurse education should contain a Common Foundation Programme where students would gain educational experience within a variety of cross-disciplinary settings enabling them to choose their later specialisation; students should receive bursaries (not grants) and nurse education should be placed within the framework of higher education.

In outlining the case for educational reform, the Judge Commission looked carefully at all the arguments in favour of maintaining the status quo and demolished them. In approaching the respected Oxford don Dr Harry Judge, the RCN also ensured both the language and the rigour of the proposals were accessible not just to nurses but also to politicians and others, who would need to be convinced the nursing profession knew unambiguously what it wanted.

Coincidentally (or not), the GNC's successor, the United Kingdom Central Council for Nursing, Midwifery and Health Visiting (UKCC), also set up a working group in 1984 from its Educational Policy Advisory Committee to review the pre-registration education of the profession. Its terms of reference were:

> 'To determine the education and training required for the profession of nursing, midwifery and health visiting in relation to the health care needs in the 1990's and beyond and to make recommendations.' (UKCC 1985a)

Over the next two years, the UKCC produced a series of nine project papers (UKCC 1985a–f; 1986a; 1987a,b) outlining its views on issues ranging from student status to the vexed question of the future of the enrolled nurse. What was striking was the degree of consensus between the Judge Commission and the various statutory bodies. The comment of White (1985), that expediency was the hallmark of the nursing profession's response to change, may have sounded cynical but it had a ring of truth about it.

In May 1986, the UKCC published *Project 2000 — A new preparation for practice* (1986b). The report contained 25 recommendations for change (see Appendix II). In essence they were:

1. A complete separation of education from service, with students having supernumerary status.
2. A Common Foundation Programme (CFP) for all students, followed by 'branching' into five areas of registration (midwifery as the fifth Project 2000 branch was later dropped at the request of midwives).
3. A practitioner who would be taught the skills to work in institutional and non-institutional settings.
4. Academic recognition would be sought for the professional qualifications of Project 2000 nurses.
5. An end to enrolled nurse training with full protection guaranteed for existing enrolled nurses.

In the summer of 1986, the UKCC launched a massive consultation and public relations exercise to ascertain the feelings of the profession towards its recommendations. Almost 1900 people wrote in with individual comments, as did approximately 600 groups involving another 8000 people. Added to this, there were the 40 formal organisations ranging from the RCN and the Confederation of Health Service Employees (COHSE) to statutory bodies like the four National Nursing Boards of the UK. Finally, there were the meetings the UKCC held over the summer months, which were attended by an estimated 30 000 to 50 000 people (UKCC 1986a). It is little wonder that a *Nursing Times* poll in October of that year found that only 22 per cent of nurses had not heard of Project 2000 (Dickson 1986).

But, while only eight per cent of respondents showed clear disapproval, only 31 per cent gave Project 2000 an unqualified approval. There was, the UKCC (1986a) acknowledged, one recurrent, overall doubt:

> 'whether sufficient political will and sufficient money and manpower (sic) will be found for change'. (p. 2)

It recognised it had a delicate path to tread. It had to assuage the concerns of those who were worried the reforms would be pushed through at any cost, as well as those who did not want to see a loss of the momentum for educational change that had gathered behind Project 2000.

At its meeting in January 1987 the UKCC agreed, in light of the feedback received during the consultation exercise, to a modified, although largely unchanged, policy on education and training reform. This was presented to ministers of the UK Health Departments on 5 February 1987 (UKCC 1987a). Considering the length of Project 2000's germination, in relative terms it did not have too long to wait for an answer.

Mindful of the sustained, negative publicity surrounding the chronic underfunding of the NHS in the early months of 1988, John Moore, the then Secretary of State for Health (England), skilfully drew much of the expected criticism of the Government by announcing its approval of Project 2000 to delighted nurses at the RCN Annual Congress in May 1988. One year later, his successor, Kenneth Clarke, announced the first wave of 13 demonstration sites to the same audience. By the summer of 1989, Project 2000 had arrived.

On reflection, it is hard to overestimate the success of nursing when compared to other professions at that time. Faced with a radical Conservative Government that was bent, it would appear, to break the power of the professions, nursing uniquely set its own agenda. As well as Project 2000, in the space of seven years, nursing succeeded in arguing for, and getting, its own independent (Pay) Review Body to settle pay awards. It also developed a clinical career structure, which, even if it was poorly managed in its implementation, offered nurses for the first time the opportunity to be rewarded for their clinical skills.

Teachers on the other hand, after a prolongd series of strikes, lost even their right to negotiate their own pay. Lawyers (Lord Chancellor's Office 1989) and doctors (Department of Health 1989) found changes being made, without their consent, to their own working practices. Only the nursing profession was able to respond to the challenges it faced internally and externally and come up with a solution. Project 2000 was not imposed on nurses, it was composed by them.

MYTHS AND REALITIES

What sort of reception did the first Project 2000 nurses receive from the profession? It would be gratifying to state they received a warm welcome from the profession, but it is clear that the response was often cool and all too frequently downright hostile (Casey 1990; Naish 1990; Dolan 1991; Clegg 1992). This section will look at some of the myths and truths that lie at the heart of Project 2000.

> 'These Project 2000 nurses are learning nursing out of a book, will go straight into education or management, because nursing patients will not be good enough for them, and they will probably take my job away when they qualify because they will have a diploma or degree and I do not.'

These views while appearing extreme, are based on the comments made to and about Project 2000 students. Yet distressing and, as will be shown, unfounded as these comments may be, they are neither original nor new. Undergraduates have been hearing them for years. When the first undergraduate nursing courses began in Scotland in 1959, the students were seen as something out of the ordinary, something different, something to watch. But given the very practical orientation of nursing, it was not long before undergraduates as a species began to be seen with a measure of mistrust. Luker (1984), herself a nurse graduate, described 'the belief which conventional nurses hold concerning the inverse relationship between intellectual dexterity. Whilst the belief has no factual foundation, it is perpetuated through the apprenticeship system where pursuit of knowledge is secondary to practical experience.' (pp. 6–7)

Undergraduates were considered too clever to be nurses, and were therefore deemed to have their own hidden agenda for coming into nursing. No one could quite work it out, but the consideration that undergraduates would come into nursing with similar values and attitudes as any other entrant (Kelly 1991) did not seem to enter the equation.

What became of graduates of nursing and are there parallels to be drawn with Project 2000? Before answering the latter half of this question, it is necessary to examine the career trajectories of the graduates themselves, for it is there many of the myths surrounding Project 2000 may be laid to rest. Each myth will be examined in turn.

'Project 2000 nurses are learning nursing out of a book'

It is true that Project 2000 nurses spend considerably more time in the classroom setting, but since they are studying at diploma and degree level, this is hardly surprising. However, there is a more fundamental issue which is all too often lost in the heat of embattled rhetoric. As Pearson (1992) points out:

'Nursing, as a collective, frequently misses the point of its very existence: the provision of a nursing service to those who need, seek, or are directed to, nursing.' (p. 213)

Although blindingly obvious, it is critical that nurses are as knowledgeable as possible in providing *informed* care to patients and clients. Benner (1984) has pointed out that:

'Experience based on skill acquisition is safer and quicker when it rests upon a sound educational base.'

If nursing theory and practice could be visualised it might be in the shape of a 'T', with the perpendicular bar representing theory and the horizontal bar practice (see Figure 1.2). For the many years that nursing students have been used and abused as 'pairs of hands' the mainstay of their learning has been practice — the horizontal bar of the 'T', with insufficient attention paid to their learning needs — the perpendicular bar. Undergraduates, historically, and now Project 2000 students, have the opportunity to deepen their knowledge base, the perpendicular bar of the 'T',

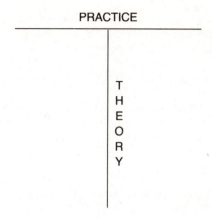

Figure 1.2 The 'T' bar of theory and practice

so they may 'uncover the knowledge embedded in clinical nursing practice' (Benner 1984).

The deeper the theory, the firmer the foundation for practice, and it is knowing why we do what we do that will enable nurses to make sense of what Schön (1987) describes as the high, safe ground of the academic institution when seen from the 'swampy lowland' that is nursing practice.

'Project 2000 nurses will go straight into management or education posts when they qualify'

This comment may bring a wry smile to the faces of graduates of nursing who confounded their critics by doing exactly the opposite of what was expected of them! Numerous studies (Marsh 1976; Kemp 1988; Hayward 1991; Winson 1993) have shown graduates stay in clinical practice out of choice. It is also worth noting where they practise. Graduates have tended to gravitate, not towards the high-tech areas of nursing, such as intensive care or casualty, but towards the high-touch areas of care, such as community, mental health, and caring for the older person. These areas are also (wrongly) considered to be Cinderella services, yet they are the very areas where the greatest levels of personal interaction and professional autonomy may be found.

Linked to the misconceptions above is the assumption that career progression means vertical mobility. Hayward (1991) has shown that many graduates have chosen to stay at the bedside and become sisters and charge nurses rather than nursing officers and tutors. This has, by and large, enabled them to retain a high degree of clinical contact and influence patient care at the point of delivery.

If the experience of graduates of nursing is anything to go by, then comparatively few Project 2000 nurses will go into education (in the traditional, institutional sense) or management. The question should not be 'why not?' but 'why should they feel a need to do so?' Clinical grading provides part of the answer, much of the rest comes from the experiences that are unfolding, copying, almost mimicking, the path that undergraduates have already travelled.

'Project 2000 nurses will take my job away when they qualify because they will have a diploma or degree and I do not'

Having a degree or diploma does not automatically make someone a good nurse. And not having one does not make someone a bad nurse either. It would be a sad reflection on the nursing profession if it only looked at the letters after a nurse's name and not the nurse as an individual.

However, as the graduates in Hayward's study showed, qualifications can also be a double-edged sword. Despite the seemingly obvious benefits to employers of having a well-educated, clinically committed workforce, a quarter of the respondents to Hayward's (1991) longitudinal study of the career paths of Kings' College nursing graduates found their degrees were perceived negatively by interview panels.

Almost inevitably, Project 2000 nurses will have to overcome the suspicion, distrust and even hostility that undergraduates faced. But much of the answer lies in the hands of Project 2000 nurses themselves. Goad (1992) suggests:

> 'Perhaps it is up to us to stand up for our rights, but this is difficult without causing some animosity.' (p. 47)

Blackburn (1992), however, is more forthright when she states:

> 'Nursing is a skill that can be taught and learned, but personality and motivation make a good nurse . . . Why then do so many still oppose Project 2000? Is it just the frightening prospect of change? If so, nurses are their own worst enemies.' (p. 45)

As Robinson shows in Chapter 3, much of the fear of the future stems from fear of change. But Ford and Jones (1992) reveal that

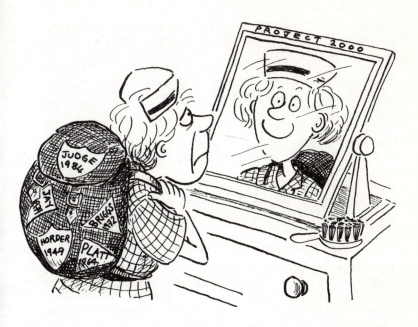

even students on conventional nursing courses share anxieties over their future. It is this group in particular who may be competing in the first instance with Project 2000 nurses for the same posts. However, Project 2000 nurses would not (or should not) get a job because they have a diploma or degree, but because they are the best candidate for the job. One can only hope that this is one area where Hayward's research about nursing graduates proves to be unfounded when the career trajectories of Project 2000 nurses are examined.

A CAREER PATTERN FOR PROJECT 2000 NURSES?

The first Project 2000 nurses completed their courses in July 1992 and it is too early to assess what career paths they may follow. However, one can speculate on what may happen. Akinsanya (1990) applies a maxim that:

> 'History teaches . . . (and) a constant reminder of the past is a prerequisite to an appreciation of its present and a prospective look at (nursing's) future.' (p. 745)

Project 2000 is a huge step forward in the education of nurses, but both Judge (1986) and Akinsanya (1990) have expressed their dismay that nursing did not fully integrate with higher education, staying, as it has, *linked to* rather than *part of* the higher education framework.

The long-term effects of this may be seen in the career trajectories of Project 2000 nurses, which may well become a hybrid of graduate and conventionally trained nurses; staying longer in practice, longer in nursing and working more frequently in the community than their conventionally trained counterparts. Unless Project 2000 courses are not only linked with, but also cemented to higher education centres, students may find themselves being sandwiched between two different educational philosophies. To paraphrase Allan (1990), newly qualified Project 2000 nurses may on one hand be expected to be frontline caregivers armed with the necessary task-oriented skills, but at the same time be expected to reflect, analyse and critique their practice — an academic exercise that does not always come naturally.

The challenge will be for Project 2000 students to promote health without losing sight of the fact that a significant amount of nursing care is delivered to people who are ill. In the 1960's the university nursing faculties in Canada changed the emphasis of their nursing curricula from psychomotor ('doing') skills to cognitive ('knowing') skills. The catalyst for these changes was a perceived transformation in society and in the delivery of health care (Love *et al.* 1989). Consequently, a decade later, employers began to notice that recent graduates seemed to be deficient in core nursing skills. If this were to be repeated with Project 2000, argues Dawes (personal communication 1991), then its future could look uncertain. A series of reports by the National Foundation for Educational Research (Leonard and Jowett 1990, Jowett *et al.* 1992) has already raised concerns.

It would be naive to assume or even hope that the biggest change to nurse education since Nightingale started recruiting 'special probationers' (Baly 1991) to train as nurses, could take place without some teething troubles. But Project 2000 represents a change that is of nursing's own making and in this sense the profession can be justifiably proud (Mason 1991).

Nonetheless, Project 2000 should not be seen to represent the pinnacle of nursing's educational achievements. It is a step in the right direction to achieving a profession that is turned on, tuned in and totally aware of its clients' needs, without losing sight of its own aspirations. While Project 2000 may not offer all the answers, it does start to address a lot more of the questions, and it is only nurses who can make it succeed. In the words of Nightingale (Baly 1991):

'No system can endure that does not march.'

REFERENCES

Akinsanya J (1990) Nursing links with higher education: a prescription for change in the 21st century. *Journal of Advanced Nursing*, **15**, 6, 744–54.

Allan C (1990) P2000 problems. *Nursing Standard*, **3**, 5, 43–4.

Baly M (1991) *As Miss Nightingale Said . . .* London: Scutari Press.

Beardshaw V (1992) *Prospects for Nursing*. In *In The Best of Health?: The status and future of health care in the UK* (eds E Beck, S Lonsdale, S Newman and D Patterson), London: Chapman & Hall.

Benner P (1984) *From Novice to Expert: Excellence and Power in Clinical Nursing Practice*. Menlo Park CA: Addison-Wesley.

Blackburn M (1992) Be proud of the project. *Nursing Standard*, **6**, 36, 44–5.

Bosanquet N (1985) Where have all the nurses gone? *Nursing Times*, **81**, 43, 16–17.

Casey N (1990) Spanning the great divide (editorial). *Nursing Standard*, **4**, 24, 3.

Clegg C (1992) P2000 Student demands fairness (letter). *Nursing Times*, **88**, 47, 12–3.

Commission on Nursing Education (1985) *The education of nurses: a new dispensation*. London: RCN. (Judge Report).

Committee of Enquiry into Mental Handicap Nursing and Care (1979). HMSO. London: Cmnd 7468 (Jay Report).

Department of Health and Social Security (1972) *Report of the Committee on Nursing*, London: HMSO Cmnd 5115 (Briggs Report).

Department of Health (1989) *Working for Patients*, London: HMSO, Cmnd 555.

Dickson N (1986) Winding up the roadshow. *Nursing Times*, **82**, 43, 47–8.

Dolan B (1991) Power to the Project? *Nursing Standard*, **5**, 28, 47.

Ford C and Jones C (1992) Students' perceptions of Project 2000. *Nursing Standard*, **6**, 33, 30–3.

Goad N (1992) Growing pains and gains. *Nursing Standard*, **6**, 36, 46–7.

Gration H M and Holland D L (1959) *The Practice of Nursing*. London: Faber.

Hayward J (1991) *Of Graduates and King's (1981–1991)*. Paper given at Eleventh Winifred Raphael Memorial Lecture. London: RCN.

Jowett S *et al.* (1992) *Introduction of Project 2000: Early Perspectives from the Students*. Slough: National Foundation for Educational Research in England and Wales.

Judge H (1986) A College Education? *Nursing Times*, **82**, 29, 31–2.

Kelly B (1991) The professional values of English nursing undergraduates. *Journal of Advanced Nursing*, **16**, 867–72.   ·

Kemp J (1988) Graduates in nursing: a report of a longitudinal study at the University of Hull. *Journal of Advanced Nursing*, **13**, 2, 281–7.

Leonard A and Jowett S (1990) *Charting the course*. A study of the 6 ENB pilot schemes in pre-registration nurse education. Slough: National Foundation for Educational Research in England and Wales.

Lord Chancellor's Office (1989) *Legal Services: A framework for the future*. London: HMSO. Cmnd 740.

Love B *et al.* (1989) Teaching psychomotor skills in nursing: a randomised control trial. *Journal of Advanced Nursing*, **14**, 11, 970–5.

Luker K (1984) Reading nursing: the burden of being different. *International Journal of Nursing Studies*, **21**, 1, 1–7.

Marsh N (1976) Summary report of a study on the career patterns of diplomates/graduates of the undergraduate course in the University of Manchester, England. *Journal of Advanced Nursing*, **1**, 6, 539–62.

Mason C (1991) Project 2000: A critical review. *Nursing Practice*, **4**, 3, 2–5.

Ministry of Health, Department of Health for Scotland and Ministry of Labour and National Service (1947) *Report of the Working Party on the Recruitment and Training of Nurses*. London: HMSO.

Naish J (1990) Project 2000 anger. *Nursing Standard*, **4**, 26, 24.

Nursing Times (1965a) Student nurses speak out. **61**, 1328.

Nursing Times (1965b) No to Platt Now. **61**, 1347.

O'Connor M (1987) The way to ward reform. *Educational Guardian*, **March 24**, 13.

Pearce C (1988) The nursing workforce. *Senior Nurse*, **8**, 3, 25–7.

Pearson A (1992) *Knowing nursing: emerging paradigms in nursing*. In *Knowledge for nursing practice* (eds K Robinson and B Vaughan). Oxford: Butterworth-Heinemann.

Robinson K and Vaughan B (1992) *Knowledge for nursing practice*. Oxford: Butterworth-Heinemann.

Royal College of Nursing (1943) *Nursing Reconstruction Committee Report*. London: RCN (Horder Report).

Royal College of Nursing (1964) *A Reform of Nurse Education: First Report of a Special Committee on Nurse Education*. London: RCN, (Platt Report).

Royal Commission on the National Health Service (1979) *Royal Commission on the National Health Service*. London: HMSO. Cmnd 7615 (Merrison Report).

Schön E (1987) *Educating the Reflective Practitioner*. Oxford: Jossey Bass.

Thomas E (1989) Graduates' careers in nursing. *Nursing Standard*, **4**, 2, 45.

UKCC (1985a) Educational Policy Advisory Committee. Project Paper 1, *Introducing Project 2000*. London: UKCC.

UKCC (1985b) Educational Policy Advisory Committee. Project Paper 2, *The Learner: Student Status Revisited!* London: UKCC.

UKCC (1985c) Educational Policy Advisory Committee. Project Paper 3, *One — Two — Three: How many levels of nurse should there be?* London: UKCC.

UKCC (1985d) Educational Policy Advisory Committee. Project Paper 4, *The Enrolled Nurse: Looking back and looking forward*. London: UKCC.

UKCC (1985e) Educational Policy Advisory Committee. Project Paper 5, *Redrawing the Boundaries?* London: UKCC.

UKCC (1985f) Educational Policy Advisory Committee. Project Paper 6, *Facing the Future*. London: UKCC.

UKCC (1986a) Project Paper 7, *The Project and the Professions: Results of the UKCC Consultation on Project 2000*. London: UKCC.

UKCC (1986b) *Project 2000: A New Preparation for Practice*. London: UKCC.

UKCC (1987a) Project Paper 8, *Counting the Cost: Is Project 2000 a Practical Proposition?* London: UKCC.

UKCC (1987b) Project Paper 9, *Project 2000: The Final Proposals*. London: UKCC.

White R (1985) *The Effects of the NHS on the Nursing Profession 1948–1961*. London: King Edward's Hospital Fund for London.

Winson G (1993) Career paths of nurse graduates. *Senior Nurse*, **13**, 1, 50–55.

CHAPTER 2

Power, Politics and Peril

John Naish

'Nursing education has fallen and seems to be imprisoned, in the trap of its own history.' (Judge 1985)

Self-perpetuation is one of the clearest hallmarks of strong, lasting professions and institutions. The profession of nursing has succeeded in retaining its essential characteristics, despite the many fundamental changes in health care that have occurred since the beginning of this century. But while this is in many ways laudable, it does mean that nursing has retained much of its bad, as well as much of its good.

Nurse training, as we shall see, had survived up till the introduction of Project 2000 largely unchanged — despite a parade of reports stretching back to the 1930's which strongly criticised the training system and urged reform. This alone is evidence of the ability of the old nursing educational system to protect and perpetuate itself. The author will explore this further later, and argue that through risking a leap into an unknown, liberal future, the profession risks a reactionary backlash from nurses socialised into loving the old certainties and from politicians who could gain significant advantage in supporting them. This reaction could be so strong as to propel the profession right back to its very educational beginnings, like a bloated sun collapsing inwards under the force of its own gravity.

SO WHAT WERE THE BEGINNINGS?

The earliest systematic training system — the Nightingale School — in 1867 created two tiers within the profession (Burnard and Chapman 1990). The school created two portals of entry; the upper, for a socially-based elite, aimed to produce the standard bearers of matron status. These nurses shouldered the hallowed mantle soon after qualifying, and by 1887, 20 of them had achieved this rank. These were the 'lady probationers'. Nurses of lower social status entered the school with their destinies firmly set — their lot was to perform the practical tasks under matron's supervision.

The core of the matron's expertise had less to do with hands-on nursing, and more to do with having the skills to ensure that matron's powerful and exalted place in the hierarchy was understood by others in the hospital.

Now look again at Project 2000. Strip away its revolutionary nature; its concern with research-based practice, the development of the knowledgeable practitioner, and the subtle divide between mechanistic tasks and hands-on nursing care. Take out all the aspects that require careful explanation before they can be understood and appreciated. Look at it through the eyes of an unsympathetic, ill-briefed non-nurse. What do we see? A two-tier system, with an educated upper tier of staff responsible for delegating work, and a less educated lower tier responsible for performing the tasks allocated to them. A little effort from those in the 'right' places could result in Project 2000 becoming grossly mutated into a modern version of nursing's earliest formal training systems.

As Dolan has pointed out in the first chapter of this book, the ideas behind Project 2000 are not new. Neither are the arguments against them. Those arguments, and the prejudices that lay behind them, successfully blocked for four decades the fundamental reform of a system that was so obviously unsatisfactory that even the anti-reformists recognised the existence of serious problems. Traditional training may have been a dinosaur, but it was a very well-adapted dinosaur when it came to one thing — survival.

Survival was the primary strength of a militarily-styled training scheme based on the unquestionable holies of rank, discipline, duty, rules, and uniformity in dress and behaviour. This historically perpetuated bullying and negativity. It inculcated disciplinarian preoccupations with the gospels of the traditional 'already-known' and concerned itself with smiting the perilously subversive 'new'. Hence the echoing chant along the Nightingale wards of 'we have always done it this way' – a mantra which promulgated the deepest suspicion of anyone who dared to break ranks.

Inculcated traditions do not die easily. The worst ones ensure that their secrets remain cloaked. Strongarm police forces, long beloved of military dictatorships, have discovered that one of the best ways of turning new recruits into torturers is to employ the simple strategy of torturing them. This way, the volunteers become so brutalised that they have no qualms about torturing others themselves — they lose respect for those who cannot withstand the pain they have borne. Project 2000's radical departure from militarist training and onto student status can look, to students who graduated from the Nursing School of Hard Knocks, to be a blow to what they believe to be the sacred pillars of their professional wisdom — and of their own self-respect.

Given the strength of this system's self-perpetuating, self-defensive mechanisms, it is a wonder that change was ever generated from within the profession itself — let alone after 40 years. In the face of all this, one can only pay tribute to those many nurses who successfully made it through the system with their ideals intact; who worked their way through the health service's often stifling management culture to a position which would enable them finally to challenge the status quo and realise their ambitions for student status.

However, the 'high-falutin' ideals of the reforms still hang by a slender thread, and it is the author's belief that now, and for the foreseeable future, they remain susceptible to debilitating contamination, if not lethal poisoning, from the diehard traditions of the old school. To illustrate Project 2000's peril further, it would be useful here to examine briefly the long and difficult labour of student status.

In 1939, a Ministry of Health Board of Education committee (Ministry of Health 1939) supported the idea of student status, albeit in a limited form, when it supported the recommendations of the General Nursing Council that nurses be allowed to study and sit preliminary examinations before entering nursing school. This move, the report suggested, would rescue new recruits from suffering the 'dual strain' of performing ward work and study. This had nothing to do with raising the profession's status. The report simply recognised the disastrous attrition rate that the traditional training system was reaping during recruits' first three months.

But when the Horder Report, established under the RCN's aegis, examined ways of implementing the 1939 report, it came down against any form of student status (Horder 1943). One can hear the distant creak of a stiff-starched cap and the stomp of a sensible shoe upon well-polished linoleum behind Horder's conclusion that:

> 'The inculcation of a sense of responsibility plays a vital part in preparing the British nurse for her career, and a course of training which turns her into a mere peripatetic observer, with no share in the life of the hospital — its trials, stresses and anxieties — must be avoided.'

However, Horder recognised that too much trial, stress and anxiety could be harmful, and called on hospitals to regulate students' workloads in accordance with their student status. As we now know, the hospitals turned a deaf ear to this. University education for nurse students was mooted in the report as a possibility for the dim distant future, but not until 'the nursing profession has put its own house in order'. Indeed. The Committee finally sat firmly on the fence, proposing a 'middle course' and stressing:

> 'There is nothing incompatible between apprenticeship and student-ship, as witness the training of engineers. The nurse trainee must, however, be a student first and an apprentice second.'

But, this was clearly not heeded. In 1948, John Cohen was so incensed by the sadistic regimes that students were having to work under that he broke away from a health committee's recommendation and produced his own *Minority report* (Cohen 1948), in which he produced a dossier of damning evidence. Cohen argued:

> 'The presence of student nurses seems to have little or no effect on the patient's length of stay . . . the independent evidence pointing to the student's preoccupation with domestic and routine duties is consistent with this result.'

And in an appendix contained in his dossier, he listed over 100 testimonies from student nurses who had dropped out from training. Today, these stories remain as stark reminders of the way in which students suffered a perpetual gamut of callous and blatant bullying at the hands of nurses in the higher rungs of the hierarchy.

One typical example came from a student who, after a long,

laborious day, was required to work half an hour extra in theatres. This consequently made her late for the compulsory nightly formal meal at the nurses' residence. She was forbidden leave to explain her reason for her delay, as this would have constituted 'answering back' to sister's admonitions for her tardiness. So instead, she was made to stand for the duration of her dinner.

Nursing at hospital level was too preoccupied with its rigid, hierarchical frigidity to bother looking forward to professional empowerment; it was too busy hardening its recruits on a diet of pettiness. And so it went on, with the profession continuing to reject any moves towards supernumerary status, such as the recommendations of the Platt Committee (Platt 1964). Thus, nursing education remained largely unreformed, except, by and large, for the osmotic effect upon nursing schools of relaxations in wider social mores throughout the post-war period. As late as 1972, the report to the Briggs Co-ordinating Committee said, partly due to financial considerations, there should be no 'radical change' in the apprenticeship status of student nurses. Student status, it suggested, should be a long-term goal (Briggs 1972).

FORMING A CONSENSUS

It was only in April 1985, with the Judge Report, commissioned by the RCN, and agreed unanimously by its members, that a true impetus for reform and student status began. The report found that the problems of student wastage and poor learning outcomes were 'not new, although they do become progressively more urgent'. Social change had accelerated in the previous two decades, leaving nurse training wobbling along the hard shoulder on its penny-farthing system. Something had to be done, and nursing took the prodigious step of deciding upon a reform that would not only bring it up to date, but would take it into the next century.

With the resounding thud of a profession leaping from a fast-splintering fence, the report declared:

'Nothing less than fundamental reform can now be effective. The changes which are proposed will appear to many to be dangerous and threatening, but should not for that reason be rejected.'

The proposed changes were in essence an embryonic Project 2000; student status and all. Already the profession was aware of the costs involved, and the report stepped in quickly to argue:

> 'A better system of education might have higher unit costs, but also
> . . . it will secure an ample supply of entrants and will be at once
> smaller and more cost-effective.'

That the impetus for reform was backed by the weight of the
profession's decision-making echelons can be seen in the speedy
progress made from launch of the Judge Report to the final UKCC
Project 2000 proposals. Seemingly all at once, reports and working
groups from the English National Board and the UK Central
Council began to tear along the same lines to reach broadly similar
conclusions. To read the history of nursing reform from its pre-
war beginnings to the advent of the Project 2000 report is to
witness a sluggish, retrograde process of proposal and frustration
— up to the point of the Judge Report. This is then followed by
what appears, in retrospect, to be a blinding flash of speed. You
would believe a bureaucracy can fly.

This is not to say that the profession was completely unified
behind the prospect of the brave new Project 2000 world.

The Confederation of Health Service Employees detected, with
some degree of prescience, some of the pitfalls of letting the
Government lay its hands on Project 2000 (COHSE 1986). It
argued that support workers could be seen by the Government as
'a cheap option', and warned against:

> 'The creation of a new aide as an attempt to dilute qualified nurse care
> and also to place practitioners in the potentially dangerous situation of
> being responsible for a group of unqualified staff which they are unable
> to supervise properly due to manpower shortages.'

Support workers, it warned, would become the new enrolled
nurse.

And while COHSE accepted supernumerary status, it rejected
bursaries or student grants in favour of a training allowance set by
the nurses' Review Body, warning: 'Student grants will always be
subject to the whims of government policy.'

This highly complex dilemma still remains — full student status at
all costs, or recognition of the contradictions inherent in the nurse
student's position? Put in its simplest terms, if nursing is to remain
the *hands-on* profession, it must, for the sake of its own arguments,
ensure that the client-centred physical focus is not lost from its
students' education. At the same time, the profession must ensure

that students are educated to be Project 2000 diplomates and graduates — not the same old products of the same old NHS system. Further, to retain academic credibility, the students must be treated as being at some distance from their NHS work duties. But to go all the way along this road would mean nursing students losing their bargaining rights and power as employees. No one said it would be easy.

This ambivalence has been, and will be, exploited to the full by politicians. Of course, any government's interest lies in part in keeping divided the country's largest workforce — in order to keep defused a potentially dangerous source of unified dissent. On the evidence of history, at least, politicians can rest assured that with a little manoeuvring, any educational changes they make in response to proposals generated within the profession will never spark a unified response.

Throughout this history, there have always been two agendas behind nursing educational reform — the professional and the political. The two have always been separate, but have found common purposes at certain points in history — both in stifling reform and introducing it. The common purpose behind (the then Health and Social Security Secretary) John Moore's RCN Congress announcement that Project 2000 would go ahead was based on a shared will to see the reforms introduced. But why did a Government committed to cutting public expenditure say that it was prepared to dig deep into its pockets for Project 2000? Did it share nursing's professional aspirations? Had it seen the light? Was it acting out of dewy-eyed philanthropy? This Conservative administration, especially during the Thatcher years, was marked for its firm stance against what it saw as professional hegemony. This can be seen in the action's of John Moore's successor, Kenneth Clarke. The caveat Mr Clarke placed in the letter he sent to the UKCC giving the go-ahead for the reforms; that enrolled nurse training should continue until support worker training was introduced into districts, indicates clearly that his priorities in introducing reform were directed not simply towards helping nurses do what they wanted (although winning grateful ovations from the profession would be no great hardship). The Government's priorities were directed instead towards maintaining hospital staffing levels into the next century.

Demography had always proved a strong spur in making the politicians and the profession look again (and again) at nurse education's sky-high wastage rates. The fact that the interests of Messrs Moore and Clarke lay in ensuring adequate *staffing* levels — not *nursing* levels — gives us a crucial insight into the Government's own motives for advancing Project 2000.

The Government's strategy was, of course, an understandably pragmatic one. The sacrifice of continuing to train nurses for the now-discontinued second-level EN registration for a few years was, at the time, criticised as unfair and immoral. But from the Government's viewpoint, this human cost must have been a comparatively small and temporary price to pay in ensuring that wards would continue to have adequate cover during the transition to Project 2000 and beyond. It would also ensure health authorities felt pushed into quickly introducing health care support worker preparation. The Government may well have worried that health authorities, bounding over with enthusiasm for introducing Project 2000 nurses — and having many nurses in their management structures — would put support worker introduction low down on their priority lists. This was not where the Government wanted it. Support workers were what it wanted — and in very large numbers.

There is, as any journalist will tell you, no such thing as a free lunch. Nursing must realise there is no such thing as a free Project 2000, and it must ask what the Government wants out of the deal. A thorough examination of the gift horse's mouth could reveal some disturbingly Trojan ancestry. Perhaps if the Government had shown its hand, and openly demanded the pay-off that it wanted in return for educational reform, the profession might have thought twice before accepting it. The author believes that the Government's undeclared deal, in terms of the cliché Victorian northern industrialist addressing his heir, would be: 'I'm not going to pay all that money to educate you in order to have you giving baths and talking to sick people all day.'

The view from the Department of Health window during the late 1980's was dominated by the demographic time bomb; by the awesome prospect of having to recruit up to half of all of the suitably qualified women coming out of school in order to maintain current NHS staffing and wastage levels. Conroy and Stidson (1988) predicted that between 1983 and 1993 there would be a 17 per cent rise in people aged over 75, and a 31 per cent drop in school leavers. They warned that the NHS was 'losing its battle to compete with other employers to recruit school leavers' — particularly those with 5 'O' levels/GCSEs and 2 'A' levels.

Any government worth its political salt would seek to circumvent such a problem. Meeting it head on would prove much too costly financially and far too risky numerically. And so, thinking laterally, the first solution would be *employ significantly fewer qualified nurses* — a solution forwarded by the above authors. This immediately sparks its own problems: who is going to care for the patients, and how will they cope with shallower founda- tions in education and training? Of course, there is also the question: how can we do it cheaper?

The answer the Government found in its reading of the proposals for Project 2000. What the politicians saw when they read between the lines of the proposals was a strategy they could develop to employ nurses as ward managers — as the link person between management and workforce — doling out the orders, dealing with the paperwork and taking professional responsibility for drug administration. Their market-based rationale would have led them to believe that this could well be acceptable to the profession in the long run. 'After all,' their thoughts would have run, 'everybody wants to better their lot, why not offer the nurses the chance to take over many of the junior doctors' roles? It would be worth it for them, and cheaper for us.'

This all fitted in well with the Government's own seamless robe of NHS reforms, where financial accountability came at the top of the priority list. It is no coincidence that at this time, Eric Caines was drafted in from his acrimonious introduction of Fresh Start, the reshuffle of prison staff's working arrangements, to head the NHS Personnel Directorate and shortly afterwards to take over respon- sibility for NHS staff training. In an interview with the author (Naish 1990), Mr Caines (who has since left the NHS) for the first time publicly laid out his intentions for nursing:

'Project 2000 will bring out highly-trained professionals who we will have to use properly,' he said. 'Nurses are locking themselves in too tight a definition. What's a doctor and what's a nurse? There's work to be done, you get the work done by the people who are best qualified to do it.' And he declared: 'Hands-on care is below nurses' level of competence. The nurse will become the overall assessor of the care that the individual needs to have (from the support workers).' In his terms, he added: 'A higher quality, cheaper service, with a competitive edge will be achieved by those who make the most improvement in their labour costs. It's just common sense.'

The extent of the radical workload reversal which Mr Caines envisaged for the profession can be ascertained from a comment he made to NHS managers, claiming nurses spend 95 per cent of their time delivering 'random care' — which should be performed by health care assistants — while they ought to be doing 'a clinical job, purely and simply' (Hart 1991). In the Cainesian scenario, from the ranks of the Project 2000 diplomates and graduates would stride the new elite, the new upper tier, the new matron, grasping selfishly at the ankles of educational reform like the horror film cliché of the hand from the grave. This new elite would hold the rod, translating the word of the hospital administrators into the practical hands-on work of the health care assistant.

Project 2000-educated nurses may not want that. The rest of the profession has openly stated, again and again, it does not want that. But someone else is paying the piper. And if nurses want to prevent this all from happening, they must pay extremely close attention to the tune that future governments will be calling. For it may propel nursing down the nebulous spiral of what it has already known and experienced — right back to square one.

Nursing does have, however, one crucial ace up its sleeve. It has Project 2000 in its hands. How it plays this card will determine the future of Project 2000 — if it is to have a future. For if the profession does not quickly start to prove that Project 2000 can work, either on its own terms or on the politicians', the results could be disastrous. Already we have witnessed hints as to the early 'sell-by' date set by the Government for the reforms — the Department of Health Nursing Officer for Education warned early in 1992 that Project 2000 funding would be threatened if the initiative did not show signs of being a success within three years (*Nursing Standard* 1992a). While Health Secretary Virginia Bottomley later attempted to dismiss this report in the Commons as the result of confusion (*Nursing Standard* 1992b) the exact source of this 'confusion' remains to be discovered.

THE COST-EFFECTIVE TWO-STEP

Governments can give, and governments can take away. Kenneth Clarke, as Health Secretary, gave the go-ahead for Project 2000's first demonstration sites. A few short years later, in 1992, Mr Clarke, as Education Secretary, demanded of the teaching profession that it destroy its own academically-orientated educational preparation and return to giving its novices hands-on classroom training. In a situation where the system was failing to produce adequately educated school-leavers, because of a multitude of intertwining socio-economic and educational factors, Mr Clarke appealed to the British voter's traditional mistrust of academia, and blamed it all on professional ivory towerism. Teaching had failed to prove value for money on the basis of its own professional aspirations. So how can nursing succeed both in having Project 2000 its way, and winning the approval of future governments for it? The profession can use the reforms to change a future government's tune, by presenting it with a song that is even sweeter to its finance-orientated ears. This tune we could call the Cost-Effective Two-Step. If the profession is truly committed to its belief in a hands-on, research-based workforce of reflective practitioners, it must prove it. It must take its argument to ministers and argue in practical terms — value for money. It must ensure it produces solid research to show that care delivered by hands-on, research-based, reflective practitioners cuts hospital length of stay, lowers readmission rates, and results in patients recovering quicker and better. Such a proof will have to be watertight. And nursing will have to be prepared to give it the full backing of all its professional resources. For when (and if) this evidence is gathered, it will sail against the running tide of prejudice. Hospital Trusts have begun their existence by looking at new ways of treating patients. And the cost-effective deals they have started to explore follow a trend which involves less, not more, skilled nurse cover. This is best exemplified by the move towards creating 'patient hotels', where patients can recuperate from operations under hospital supervision, but under the care of staff who are not qualified nurses. Hospital administrators will have to be presented forcefully with strong arguments before they are convinced by nurses that they have taken the completely wrong tack.

A great deal of responsibility weighs, therefore, on the shoulders of the cohorts entering nursing during Project 2000's formative years. These students, who must sometimes feel like guinea pigs, must remember that their true destiny is to overrun the lab. Throughout their college years, they will have to defend the purity of their education against dilution by nurses who will want to teach them to practise the way they were taught, rather than 'doing all that stuff they teach at College' — a subject Jill Robinson covers in detail in Chapter 3. For many existing staff, to admit the new training is better without feeling professionally obsolete will prove a difficult mental contortion to achieve. The UKCC's Post-Registration and Practice initiative (UKCC 1990) could hopefully ameliorate this situation for staff who believe that:

'For those who nurse, our nursing is a thing which, unless we are making progress every year, every month, every week, take my word for it we are going back.' (Baly 1991)

The new cohorts will also have to survive the continuing fall-out from Project 2000's massive reorganisation of schools of nursing into higher educational institutions. They must quickly learn to act as adult higher education students; to give time and support to their tutors, who themselves have a great deal to learn and cope with in this transitional phase — as Jan Charlwood explains in Chapter 4. Furthermore, students will somehow have to deal with a chronic underfunding of library resources which may for years continue to threaten to strangle the new professionalism at its research-based academic roots (Shepherd 1992). Research among the first English Project 2000 courses has shown that pressure from students for more resources can result in extra library funding from colleges (Shepherd and Yeoh 1990).

When the first cohorts themselves become newly-qualified staff on the wards, they will have to continue to defend Project 2000, working to ensure that diplomate research takes root in the remaining barren ground of blinkered professional areas. They must resist the attrition of colleagues' and non-nurses' prejudices and remain in large numbers in hands-on nursing. The ghost of 'all those Project 2000 lot are going to do is go straight into management' must be exorcised from within the profession itself before the case for pure Project 2000 can successfully be taken to Government. Then, once the new cohorts have established their regime, they will have to prove that it works better. And all this must be achieved before either Project 2000 becomes politically hijacked, or the health service is transformed so radically that nursing is rendered unable to prove itself.

When, and if, these pioneers prove the wisdom of high quality care delivered by educated qualified nurses, they should finally have run out of opponents.

REFERENCES

Baly M (1991) *As Miss Nightingale Said . . .* London: Scutari Press.

Briggs (1972) Co-ordinating Committee Working Group II, report to the Co-ordinating Committee, London: HMSO.

Burnard P and Chapman C (1990) *Nursing Education: the Way Forward.* London: Scutari Press.

Cohen J (1948) Ministry of Health, Department of Health for Scotland, Ministry of Labour and National Service, *Working Party on the Recruitment and Training of Nurses, the Minority Report.* London: HMSO.

Commission on Nursing Education (1985) *The education of nurses, a new dispensation.* London: RCN. (Judge Report).

Confederation of Health Service Employees (1986) *Response to the UK Central Council for Nurses, Midwives and Health Visitors.* Banstead: COHSE.

Conroy M and Stidson M (1988) The Black Hole (population changes and the implications for the NHS labour market). *Health Manpower Management,* **14**, 3, 6–9.

Hart E (1991) Ghost in the Machine. *Health Service Journal,* **101**, 5281, 20–22.

Ministry of Health Board of Education (1939) *Interdepartmental Committee on Nursing Services, Interim Report.* London: HMSO.

Naish J (1990) Vision or Nightmare? *Nursing Standard,* **5**, 12, 18–19.

Nursing Standard (1992a) Funding is dependent on success of Project 2000. *Nursing Standard,* **6**, 19, 8.

Nursing Standard (1992b) News. *Nursing Standard,* **6**, 21, 11.

Royal College of Nursing (1943) *Nursing Reconstruction Committee.* London: RCN. (Horder Report).

Royal College of Nursing (1964) *A reform of nurse education.* London: RCN. (Platt Report).

Shepherd T (1992) P2000 — read all about it. *Nursing Standard,* **6**, 22, 41.

Shepherd T and Yeoh J (1990) *Resourcing Project 2000 Nursing Courses — the Role of Library and Information Services.* London: RCN.

United Kingdom Central Council for Nursing, Midwifery and Health Visiting (1990) The report of the Post-Registration Education and Practice Project. London: UKCC.

CHAPTER 3

All Change — Project 2000's Greatest Challenge

Jill E Robinson

'Now there are opportunities for nursing to take control over its own destiny.' (Casey 1993)

INTRODUCTION

Project 2000 (UKCC 1986) heralds fundamental changes in the United Kingdom on several fronts, not only in the way nurses are educated but also in the way they will practise in the future. Some degree of resistance to these changes may be inevitable if one looks to the way growth has been received by the profession in the past, and is already emerging in the form of increased stress, anxiety and ambivalence towards Project 2000, both within the profession and in other allied disciplines.

Historically, any major change has been hard won in the face of powerful stereotypical images of nursing which have acted as bridle and bit to the galloping creativity of individuals within the profession. Some of the problems which Project 2000 attempts to address are not new and have emerged time and again in various forms. Examples of these can be found in both the attempts to challenge the traditional role and status of nurses in relation to other professional groups, and also in attempts to articulate the nature of nursing and its unique body of knowledge.

This chapter draws on data from a three-year local evaluation of Project 2000 to juxtapose the rhetorical descriptions of the aims of Project 2000 with participants' descriptions of their own experiences. It uses Peter Marris' work (1984) on loss and change to provide a theoretical framework for understanding the processes involved where evidence of resistance to change has been found and to inform some ideas about how such resistance might be managed.

STATUS ISSUES

The growing body of literature pertaining to Project 2000 suggests that one of its central aims is to contribute to raising the status of nursing in relation to other professional groups. Previous attempts to challenge traditional views of the role and status of nurses have had limited effect.

The Briggs Report (DHSS 1972), in its exploration of how members of the profession saw themselves, found that the nurse's role was still seen by many as 'handmaiden to the doctor'.

This has continued to be an issue in nursing and is vividly portrayed by Muff (1982) in her paper *Handmaiden, battleaxe, whore*. She cites one doctor's comments about nurse educators changing trained nurses 'from members of a humanitarian profession to a bunch of self-seekers who are educated beyond the point of usefulness'. In her literature review of images of the nurse, Bridges (1990) notes that 'on the whole, nurses have remained unassertive and submissive despite enormous developments in their own specialist role'.

Several authors have also drawn attention to the relationship between the status of nursing as a predominantly female occupation and the status of women and women's knowledge *per se* (Hagell 1989; Chandler 1991; Gordon 1991).

Some concern about the status of nursing has roots in the more recent past. Nightingale's earliest work (1860) was clearly focused on administering health services, and the efficiency of hospital administration became almost the exclusive domain of senior nurses in their role as matron. Management and administration remained primarily the responsibility of nurses until the early 1980's when the Griffiths Report (DHSS 1983) disempowered senior nurses by introducing to health services the concept of general management. The cost of general management to the nursing profession in terms of power and status were enormous. Akinsanya (1990) argues that 'recent health services reorganisations have succeeded in destroying the managerial confidence which the nursing profession has built up over the years to a point of total loss to the profession';

and Gibbs *et al.* (1991) talks of

'the process whereby senior nurses were sidestepped and stripped of their power during the structural changes in the British National Health Service (NHS) following the Griffiths' Report'.

Although progress appears to have been made in the way nurses relate to the medical profession and vice versa (Porter 1991) the role and status of nurses is quite evidently still an issue for Project 2000, of which a primary aim is to increase the professional status of the nurse in relation to other health care professionals and assist the acquisition of skills needed for more autonomous practice (*Senior Nurse* 1987). Supernumerary status aims to challenge the perpetuation of a submissive, compliant workforce by attempting to protect the student from the socialising influences of workplace culture (Bowman 1989) and by achieving academic credibility it attempts to put nurses on a more equal footing with other health professionals.

THE NATURE OF NURSING

The notion of what attributes and functions contribute to the role of the nurse has its roots in the distant past. This notion is held and maintained by the profession itself and also by the society in which nursing takes place. There is a wide understanding by both nurses and members of the general public about the meaning of what it is to be a nurse and to be nursed.

Farr and Moscovici (1984) use the term 'social representation' to describe those collectively held beliefs, emotions, images and ideas 'which are related to a particular mode of understanding and of communicating — a mode which creates both reality and common sense'. The collective, public image of nursing can therefore be seen as a social representation built from past experiences rather than from the reality of current practice and the needs of the future.

This representation or image of nursing is summarised thus in the Briggs Report (DHSS 1972):

'nursing retains an image which belongs to the late nineteenth century. "The lady with the lamp" or the "ministering angel" and similar visions linger in the mind.'

Nurses, it states, are nearly always seen as women; special, dedicated and disciplined women. Orr (1990) comments:

'While the Briggs Committee report was published in 1972, it still rings true today. Perhaps the traditionalism of nursing is resistant to all major change?'

Alternatively, its currency could be attributed to a fundamental paradox. At one level, the level of social representation, everyone knows what nursing is — or rather they know what kind of people nurses are. At the same time, but at a different level, even nurses themselves have extraordinary difficulty when it comes to describing what is special about nursing when required to identify and protect their professional boundaries. At the collective level, the nature of nursing is understood more in terms of who nurses are whereas at the professional level the focus is on what nurses do that separates them from other groups. The difficulty in articulating a theory of practice has roots which can be traced back to the notion of nursing as common-sense women's work supported to some extent by Nightingale herself with her claim that 'every woman is a nurse' (Nightingale 1860, in Akinsanya 1990).

This difficulty also relates to nursing's historical dependency on the medical profession for its knowledge base, research and focus for practice (Hagell 1989) and its neglect for nursing theory (Hogan and DeSantis 1991).

The answer may well be found in developing a community of nurse practitioners who can not only understand a coherent theory of practice but also continually contribute to its development. Such theory will only develop as nurses increasingly engage in researching their own practice.

Much has been written and said about the need for nursing to become research based. That there is still limited good nursing research may, in part, be due to resistance to the notion of the academic nurse. It may be, on the other hand, that most practising nurses have only limited opportunities to acquire the necessary skills, academic support and funding to carry out quality research. The move towards higher education is perhaps the missing ingredient that might move research based practice out of the realms of rhetoric and into the heart of the everyday world of nursing practice. The continuing development of a substantive theory of nursing depends on the profession's wholesale ability to subject its emergent theory to academic debate. In order to participate in this debate the nursing community must be enabled, through education, to provide a critical, knowledgeable and empowered audience to scrutinise the work of its researchers and academics. Project 2000 doesn't just address the content of this debate but actually seeks to elevate it by raising the academic level of the qualification which nurses receive at the end of their nursing course. Higher education aims also to enable us to articulate what we do and why we do it for an external audience that, in a climate of Health Care Assistants and skill mix negotiation, may well become increasingly sceptical about the value of professional nursing.

Although opinion differs as to whether or not Project 2000 is the most appropriate vehicle for change, few in the nursing profession would deny the importance of maintaining continuous progression in order to meet the changing health care needs of the future. Florence Nightingale, with extraordinary vision, warned

'For we who nurse, our nursing is a thing which, unless in it we are making progress every year, every month, every week take my word for it we are going back.' (Abel-Smith 1960)

Current work researching the impact of Project 2000 (Robinson 1991a) indicates the emergence of areas of resistance from both educators and practitioners to some aspects of Project 2000. This has led to a return to the work of Peter Marris (1984) to try to provide a theoretical underpinning to the processes of resistance that are evidencing themselves, and to raise some cautionary comments that can be made in relation to the way Project 2000 is being implemented.

THE PSYCHOLOGY OF CHANGE

Marris (1984), in his study of the effects of loss and change on different groups of people, describes what he calls 'the conservative impulse'. He defines this as a characteristic ambivalence to change which is a necessary precursor to adaptation to anything new. He also suggests resistance to new ideas is more profound than simple prejudice and class interest and is as necessary to survival as our ability to adapt. The physical environment in which we live has to be seen as predictable in order that we may understand our behaviour and the behaviour of others within it. In order to adapt to change, we must have a system by which we can place the new in the context of the old and familiar. Where the physical world is unpredictable, human beings will impose a system upon it using the ability to extract underlying laws from events in order to make sense of the world. Even when experiences do not fit the construed system, they will be ignored or avoided rather than allowed to undermine the validity of the system.

Of particular interest to the issue addressed in this chapter is Marris' suggestion that the construction of meaningful perceptions is a cumulative process. Our system for making sense of the world is built slowly, layer upon layer, from early childhood and throughout adult life. The revision of principles which have their foundations in the distant past and by which so much of the past has been interpreted is a much more arduous and impenetrable task than that of making events conform to past principles.

Resistance to the fundamental changes encompassed by Project 2000 can therefore be understood in terms of the extent to which those changes undermine the collective image of what nursing should be about, and the need to make the differing health care needs that are emerging in our society conform to past principles for meeting those needs.

How, therefore, does Marris account for the fact that people do eventually manage to adapt to all kinds of change in their lives and, more specifically, that the nursing profession has eventually responded positively to fundamental changes in its past? Marris suggests that although conservatism is necessary for survival, in that mastery of the environment rests on being able to abstract regularities from unique events, reaction to change need not always be defensive. He maintains that the conservative impulse is not incompatible with growth as long as the 'thread of continuity' is not broken and a return to an earlier stage for reassurance is still possible. An example of this can be found within the nursing profession in the continued use of the term 'sister' which is a clear reflection of nursing's religious, vocational origins (Abel-Smith 1960).

It is through these 'threads of continuity' that the growth of collective endeavour, such as the development of a profession, can evolve from generation to generation, protecting the individual's need to make sense of the new by reference to the past.

PROJECT 2000: A NEW PREPARATION FOR PRACTICE

As described in the previous chapters, Project 2000 attempts to facilitate necessary changes within the profession by making a number of fundamental changes to the way nurses are educated simultaneously and in one main effort. These changes include a major change in emphasis which now requires students to place the concept of ill health firmly within the context of normality and well-being. Notions of holistic, individualised care replace the malfunctioning machine concepts inherent within the medical model.

Project 2000 also aims to move the focus of health care to a range of settings, challenging the notion that nursing takes place primarily in a hospital environment. The introduction of supernumerary status for students aims to de-emphasise the students' service-giving role in order to meet the educational needs of the student rather than the service needs of the organisation. Finally, academic skills are to be developed, valued and rewarded with a Diploma/ Degree in Nursing or Higher Education.

These changes necessarily challenge fundamental aspects of a traditional view of what nursing is and who nurses are. The compliant, willing, caring and dedicated angel who has no career ambitions (Bridges 1990) is replaced by the flexible, adaptable, critically analytic and autonomous practitioner who is well able to relate intelligently and assertively with other health care professionals.

EXPLORING LOCAL ISSUES OF RESISTANCE

During the initial phase of the evaluation research that is taking place within the Suffolk and Great Yarmouth College of Nursing and Midwifery, in partnership with the Suffolk College, key areas of change were explored in terms of participants' experiences of the implementation of Project 2000 (Robinson 1991a). Initial key person interviews broadly confirmed the national vision of the aims of Project 2000 (UKCC 1986; *Senior Nurse* 1987) with minor variations to reflect local aspirations. Questionnaires were distributed to teachers, clinical staff and students from the first two intakes of the Diploma of Higher Education (Nursing) course throughout 1990.

These questionnaires were exploratory in intent and generated primarily qualitative data which were to be used to illuminate our understanding of the experiences of both staff and students of the early stages of Project 2000 implementation. A total of 25 question-naires were returned from teaching staff, 78 from students and 54 from clinical staff. The findings from this phase of the study have been published elsewhere (Robinson 1991b, 1992) but evidence of resistance to change was beginning to emerge to some extent across all data sets.

Although there were some very positive trends throughout the data sets, including a distinct thread of optimism and commitment to the vision of Project 2000, data collected especially from students show a concern about aspects of the course which present the most fundamental challenges to their beliefs about nursing. For example, although students were intellectually prepared for a curriculum which moves from a community, health, normality perspective to a hospital, ill-health perspective, the majority of students who responded to the questionnaire expressed an almost desperate need to get involved with 'real patients' on 'proper wards' early in their course. They tended not to feel like 'proper nurses' in placements outside the hospital environment and appeared to be concerned about the relevance of these placements to nursing.

The following examples illustrate this range of feeling:

> 'my GP laughed when he heard that going to work in Asda for a week will help me become a nurse. I feel this attitude of regarding Project 2000 as a joke is widespread no matter how much the teachers tell you it isn't.'

> 'I thought I would have some practical experience during the early part of my course such as bed making — some of our group have been auxiliary nurses and so I feel that I am at a disadvantage to them.'

> 'At the moment, a lot of us feel we are never going to get on the wards and our motivation is getting low.'

Staff in clinical areas also appeared to share a notion of real nursing being to do with hospitals and patients in bed. Practical experience was often described only in terms of ward experience and similar emphasis was placed by many on early ward-based placements. As one nurse states:

> 'I believe the students are not introduced to the ward environment at an early enough stage in their training — the students still need equal practical preparation.'

Although students have considerable contact with the community in their first year, including the community nursing service, another nurse claims that

> 'for the first year of their training they have little contact with nursing in a practical sense.'

The concept of supernumerary status also attracted a range of comments. Some of the qualified nurses who responded to questions about supernumerary status expressed positive views which they related to their own experiences of being part of the workforce during training. One nurse spoke of being 'the workforce on extremely busy wards' and 'after each shift you have to make time for your own private study'. Several saw the advantages of this concept in terms of better supervision, 'less pressure', 'more time to question and challenge existing practice' and 'time to learn properly and not as part of the working team'.

A tendency towards resistance, however, could also be found in some of the reactions of both students and staff to the notion of supernumerary status. There appeared to be some evidence that both clinical staff and some students expected to 'work shifts' rather than negotiate their times of work to meet educational needs. There also appeared to be some discomfort with the role of supernumerary students, with many students expressing feelings of alienation because they were not treated as part of the service teams.

> 'On the whole, staff were very friendly but did not really know what to do with us.'

> 'I think they are having problems coping with us being supernumerary. They're not quite sure what to do with us.'

> 'Enrolled nurses very often offered to help the qualified nurse so that I was left to watch, I felt like a spare part a lot of the time.'

This was occasionally reflected in the responses of clinical staff as illustrated in the following example,

> 'The students feel totally alien to the team and a spare part. I think they feel "in the way", apart from getting bored silly.'

On the whole, clinical staff presented a fairly accurate account of the nature of supernumerary status with comments such as 'being able to learn and observe and apply what you learn in the classroom in a practical setting without being counted as part of the routine workforce.'

'Not using the student as cheap labour, or as just a pair of hands but involving them to learn only.'

Questions about what students are actually expected to do on placements, however, elicited a wide range of responses suggesting that although many people know what it means, its practical interpretation varies considerably.

The relationship between higher education and quality of care has been explored by Luker (1984) who refers to 'the belief which conventional nurses hold concerning the inverse relationship between intellectual ability and manual dexterity'.

The notion, inherent in Project 2000, that nurses should acquire academic skills in order to enhance their ability to practise was another area where resistances appeared to be emerging from the data gathered from students and staff in clinical areas.

Although some students saw the value of acquiring academic skills, several felt it would be at the expense of learning 'real' nursing skills.

'In my opinion, you learn from experience, not from text book theories . . . I feel I shall come out from this course with a high degree of knowledge about personality and the self etc., but I shall have no practical or useful skills necessary to nursing.'

'Nurses, no matter what the style of training, ultimately have to be practical carers and not people who may be very clever academically but practically will make terrible nurses.'

Clinical staff again showed a varied response to the value of gaining academic skills. Some expressed a personal need for a more academic training,

'when I first started my training I really felt frustrated at the amount of hands on work compared to classroom experience. I am sure I am not alone in feeling that I was capable of much more academic input than was offered in the past',

and others saw its value in relation to improving practice,

'I feel it will benefit the whole profession if our actions are based on research, and will enable some of us to devote time to look into clinical practice.'

Several, however, remained unconvinced of the need to develop academic skills.

'Hands on experience is where I learned most, not from classroom or watching others.'

'I do believe too much emphasis is put on academic qualifications and not enough on practical issues.'

Data from teaching staff were less likely to include descriptions of overt resistance to the concepts inherent in Project 2000. Teachers however seemed somewhat more likely to describe their affective response to the process of change and its impact on their working experiences.

Their data, which were collected very early in the study, made frequent reference to feelings of loss of personal control, 'I feel totally out of control of the situation', 'too many variables to control'; being deskilled, 'having to mark assignments when one is not completely *au fait* with what has been taught', 'it challenges my experience and knowledge in a way that leaves me feeling deskilled'; uncertainty about the future, 'I am not sure we will produce in the end what we set out to produce' and pointed to underlying feelings of loss associated with the implementation of Project 2000. For many teachers, even those who welcomed Project 2000 with positive optimism, the reality of its early implementation for many meant a working world turned upside-down with little direction and considerable confusion. There was a consequent loss of meaning to working roles, loss of stability and a diminishing sense of personal value. It may well be that these experiences were inevitable given the extent of the changes proposed by Project 2000, coupled with extensive change and reorganisation in most other areas of health care delivery. They do, in any case, indicate a context which, according to Marris (1984), would provide fertile ground for the kind of resistance that has already been described and which might act as a potential source of anxiety and frustration for educators who see their vision distorted by the reactionary attitudes of clinical staff, teachers and students alike.

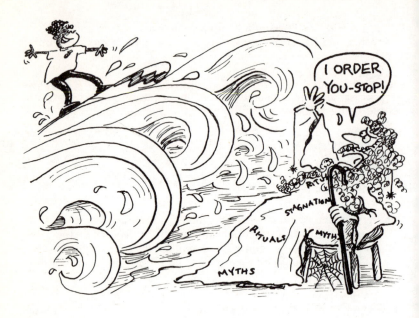

IMPLICATIONS

Marris (1984) presents us with an alternative way of understanding these trends. Is it not possible that these areas of resistance provide the 'threads of continuity' through which professional development and change can take place? Project 2000 is a radical challenge to a widely held image of nursing, with many of our current practices built slowly and cumulatively upon principles which have their roots in the distant past. When confronted with a world in which many feel deskilled and disempowered, it is not surprising that we feel the need to hold on to some of the things that were part of a world in which our skills had obvious currency.

Although supernumerary status for students changes traditional relationships in practice situations, it can be rendered somewhat more manageable and benign by maintaining shiftwork patterns where possible. The apparent emphasis on the supremacy of the development of practical skills over the development of skills of enquiry ensures the continuing credibility of existing staff, even in a context which increasingly demands greater ability to adapt rather than to learn new skills at every point of service development.

These resistance strategies that adhere to the old in defiance of the new may well function to control the tide of change while the profession collectively takes time to re-assess the system by which it makes sense of its practices, values and beliefs. What is said about Project 2000 may well be different from what people are actually doing with it in the realities of practice-based learning. The issue of most importance, therefore, is not so much how to stop people using resistance strategies but rather to distinguish those strategies that are inherently detrimental to standards of care from those which temporarily seek to impose a familiar system on a seemingly unpredictable nursing world.

It is evident again from the data collected from teachers that what teachers felt they most needed throughout the process of implementation was more time, not just for preparation but also to reflect on and adjust to the new demands created by Project 2000. The need to use this time to re-establish a sense of meaning and cohesiveness in what teachers do is vividly illustrated by one teacher's comment:

> 'The speed of implementation of the curriculum has produced an unstable monster; an enormous alien thing.'

Other teachers ask for:

> 'a structured slot to abreact and exchange views and opinons' or 'time out at regular intervals to reflect on what has happened, is happening and be able to plan more effectively for what is to happen in the future'.

Similar evidence is emerging from a small local study which is exploring the potential development needs of new staff nurses who will have had a different kind of education from those who have been recruited in the past (Robinson *et al.* 1992). Both trained staff and students foresee the need for formally organised times to talk about differences and share common experiences if the work of nursing teams is not to be inhibited by feelings of resentment, hostility and prejudice.

The implementation of Project 2000 has provided limited opportunity for staff in both education and service to use these kinds of strategies to assist adaptation. In these circumstances, resistance strategies may well be called upon to halt the onslaught of change while new systems are developed by which they can be better understood.

CONCLUSION

In the light of Marris' work (1984), it is possible that this resistance to change is not indicative of professional intransigence but rather of an incomplete process of adaptation. With the speed at which implementation took place in the author's college, the need to retain some aspects of a more familiar predictable system may well serve to sustain meaning in a constantly changing professional world that, for many, appears chaotic, unpredictable and threatening.

This need, and the open expression of ambivalence and resistance, should not only be tolerated but also, perhaps, be actively encouraged in order to facilitate, over time, the transition from one system of beliefs to another.

It may be worth noting at this point in the argument that the creation of an internal market from strategies described in the Government's White Paper *Working for Patients* may inhibit the necessary expression of feelings of resistance. Not only do organisations need to present the best possible face to their potential customers with the appearance of a unified workforce all looking forward to the challenge of the 1990's with excitement and enthusiasm, but the emerging climate of industrial secrecy between institutions who are now potential competitors, may further limit the opportunity to balance internal experiences of change with the wider perspective of experiences of other organisations. The recent emergence of 'confidentiality clauses' in contracts awarded to staff in some trusts points to further problems in relation to the open expression of ambivalence and resistance across institutional boundaries. Wright (1992) suggests

> 'confidentiality is not being used in the best interests of patients, but as a weapon to suppress nurses when they choose to publicise their concerns about poor standards of patient care.'

This kind of activity brings the issue of confidentiality out of the realms of ethics and into the arena of internal markets and industrial secrecy with the potential danger that 'confidentiality' will be reinterpreted from a means of protecting patients to a means of protecting the interests of the organisation.

In order to maintain professional growth, nurse managers, educators and those at the highest levels of general management need not only to avoid sweeping resistances under the carpet but also to ensure that ideas continue to be exchanged and shared across a national network.

The main thrust of this argument, therefore, is that where resistance occurs it should not necessarily be perceived as a negative force within the process of change. It should, rather, be examined for its function in terms of coping with and finding meaning in a rapidly changing nursing world. It may well be that the maintenance of some aspects of traditional nursing is not a fundamental threat to the vision of nursing encompassed by Project 2000, but rather a necessary precursor to wholesale professional growth.

REFERENCES

Abel-Smith B (1960) *A History of the Nursing Profession*. London: Heinemann.

Akinsanya J A (1990) Nursing links with higher education: a prescription for change in the 21st century. *Journal of Advanced Nursing*, **15**, 6, 744–54.

Bowman G and Thompson D (1989) Key areas of change needed in nursing. *Nursing Standard*, **3**, (21), 25–27.

Bridges J M (1990) Literature review on the images of the nurse and nursing in the media. *Journal of Advanced Nursing*, **15**, 850–4.

Casey N (1993) Verve, vision and vitality. *Nursing Standard*, **7**, 18, 3.

Chandler J (1991) Reforming nurse education 1 — the reorganisation of nursing knowledge. *Nurse Education Today*, **11**, 2, 83–8.

Department of Health and Social Security (1972) *Report of the Committee on Nursing*. London: HMSO. (Briggs Report)

Department of Health and Social Security (1983) *National Health Service Management Inquiry*. London: DHSS. (Griffiths Report)

Farr R M and Moscovici S (1984) *Social Representations*. Cambridge: Cambridge University Press.

Gibbs I *et al.* (1991) Skill mix in nursing: a selective review of the literature. *Journal of Advanced Nursing*, **16**, 2, 242–9.

Gordon S (1991) Fear of caring: the feminist paradox. *American Journal of Nursing*, **February**, 45–8.

Hagell E (1989) Nursing knowledge: women's knowledge. A sociological perspective. *Journal of Advanced Nursing*, **14**, 3, 226–33.

Hogan N and DeSantis L (1991) Development of substantive theory in nursing. *Nurse Education Today*, **11**, 167–71.

Luker K A (1984) Reading nursing: the burden of being different. *International Journal of Nursing Studies*, **21**, 1, 1–7.

Marris P (1984) *Loss and Change*. London: Routledge & Kegan Paul.

Muff J (1982) *Socialisation, Sexism and Stereotyping. Women's Issues in Nursing*. St Louis: C V Mosby.

Nightingale F (1860) *Notes on Nursing: What it is and What it is not*, 2nd edn. London: Harrison & Sons.

Orr J G (1990) Tradition v Project 2000 — something old something new. *Nurse Education Today*, **10**, 1, 58–62.

Porter S (1991) A participant observation study of power relations between nurses and doctors in a general hospital. *Journal of Advanced Nursing*, **16**, 728–35.

Robinson J E (1991a) *The First Year — Experiences of a Project 2000 Demonstration District.* Ipswich: Suffolk and Great Yarmouth College of Nursing and Midwifery.

Robinson J E (1991b) Evaluating the courses. *Nursing Times,* **87**, 21, 29–30.

Robinson J E (1992) Project 2000 in practice. *Nursing Times,* **88**, 40, 28–30.

Robinson J E, Rex S and Boreman L (1992) *Exploring the Potential Impact of Project 2000 on Local Staff Nurse Development Programmes.* A study in progress commissioned by The Acute Unit, Ipswich Hospital, Ipswich.

Senior Nurse (1987) The final proposals. *Senior Nurse,* **7**, 2, 12–17.

UKCC (1986) *Project 2000: A New Preparation for Practice.* London: UKCC.

Wright S (1992) The case for confidentiality. *Nursing Standard,* **6**, 19, 52–3.

CHAPTER 4

The Challenge of Higher Education

Jan Charlwood

'Education is what survives when what has been learnt has been forgotten.'
(Skinner 1964)

Nurse education has long been under scrutiny, and much of the responsibility for enabling change placed, rightly, in the hands of the educators. Birch (1975) suggests:

> 'there appears to be a need for nurse tutors to broaden their whole outlook and to take their place within the total orbit of education in its widest sense.'

Project 2000 has given nurse teachers the opportunity to take up that challenge by encouraging the development of nurse education within an academic setting. It recommended schools of nursing should make links with higher education, and that courses should be validated jointly by both academic and professional bodies (UKCC 1986). Since such courses would be at certificate or diploma level, it was proposed that teachers would be required to hold at least a first degree. This proposal was taken up by the ENB (1989) which stated that in future all teachers of nursing should be of graduate status.

In achieving the recommendations of Project 2000, the status of nurse education has been fundamentally changed within a very short time. Already many schools of nursing have become colleges under the auspices of universities or other higher education establishments. Nursing students have been granted student status, and are encouraged to participate in the academic and social opportunities now open to them. The demand for a graduate teaching force has also exposed many more nurse teachers to the experience of higher education, thus enabling them to foster this new culture.

However, it is in the nature of challenge that it brings with it a degree of stress. Such innovations in education put great pressure on teachers, and may also be accompanied by some resistance to change, itself a source of stress and anxiety (Robinson 1991). For many teachers, the need to achieve graduate status has simply added to the high levels of anxiety they were already experiencing at this time of change. Some have obtained degrees because they were under pressure to do so, rather than to achieve any personal ambition. Many have had to undertake part-time degree courses, while still fulfilling the requirements of work and family. Very few have had the luxury of spending three full years participating in the experience of university life.

Consequently, most teachers have achieved degree status at great cost to themselves, and have been denied the opportunity to absorb fully the academic culture. They are then in the invidious position of wishing to impart the ideals of higher education to their students, without having been given the chance to enjoy these for themselves.

A DIFFERENT ETHOS

Higher education has a great deal more to offer than the simple acquisition of knowledge. Moving nursing into this orbit has required a change in the aims and expected outcomes of education, as well as in the depth and breadth of the curriculum (Birchenall 1991; Chandler 1991). This will entail changes in styles of teaching, and in the role expectations of students and teachers. Because it will expose students to a new social and cultural experience, they will behave differently to traditional learners, and may be less quickly assimilated into the world of nursing.

Such changes to nurse education have all been the subject of criticism, and have therefore been a source of stress for students on the new courses. They also make increased demands on teachers, and create difficulties which need to be recognised and addressed. It is hoped that by exposing student nurses to the ethos of higher education, the culture of nurse education will change, and eventually the profession of nursing itself. The challenge then remains with those of us who teach nurses to facilitate and celebrate such change, rather than to resist it because of the problems it poses for us.

Project 2000 courses devote more time to theoretical study than traditional courses, and therefore enable students to pursue subjects in greater depth. Providing students with a sounder knowledge base in this way can, in itself, be unsettling for teaching staff. In the past, nurse tutors have tended to be generic teachers; they could teach most aspects of the curriculum, and knew more than their students did. The goal was for students to acquire a qualification, not for them to achieve parity with their teachers.

Now, on a diploma course, students may well become more knowledgeable than their teachers in many aspects of the curriculum. Subjects such as sociology, psychology and even biosciences are often taught by academics from these fields rather than by nurses, and are covered in greater depth than ever before.

Nurse teachers are learning to specialise (Birchenall 1991). They need also to feel confident that their expertise is of value, that it is no longer necessary to hold on to all aspects of the curriculum, nor to maintain credibility by apparent omniscience. It has been suggested that

> 'nurse teachers control the learning environment as rigidly as they do because they realise that their legitimacy is tenuous in the eyes of both learner and trained nurses.' (Gott 1983)

However, as education changes, it is important that teachers learn to feel comfortable about letting go, and relinquishing some of the power in the learning situation. If we are truly 'educating' our students, we should be not only 'leading out', but leading further. Our goal should be for our students to overtake us, and it should be recognised that this is not a threat but a reward.

Empowering students in this way requires confident teachers, and concerns about legitimacy and credibility need to be explored. Such anxieties may be engendered by 'the gap between theory and practice . . . universally recognised as a major problem' (Salvage 1985), and by the lack of value given to those actively involved in the practice of nursing. Teachers have little time in which to maintain close links with clinical areas, to continue to use their nursing skills and to keep in touch with changes in practice. Consequently it can be difficult for their teaching to be grounded in what is realistic, or always to take into account current innovations. It is important that these concerns are addressed, and one way forward may be the development of more posts linking education with practice. Joint appointments, in which a teacher's role is divided between a college of nursing and a clinical area, and lecturer–practitioner posts, in which a nurse has clinical and management responsibilities together with a teaching role, have been developed for these reasons (Vaughan 1989). Whilst there are enormous difficulties for the nurse attempting to combine several roles in this way, such posts offer a way of emphasising the value of clinical practice, and enabling teachers to maintain professional credibility. As long as education and practice remain divorced, there is a danger that the skilled practitioner will continue to be undervalued, and the theory–practice gap will be preserved. Moreover, teachers become starved of patient contact and deprived of the opportunities to use and develop their own skills and abilities.

Besides concerns raised about the difference between what is taught and what is practised, there have been criticisms about the increased academic content of Project 2000 courses. It has been traditional to lament that nursing is a practical job and can only be learned at the bedside, but fortunately many nurses would now agree with Benner (1984) that

> 'the person with limited background knowledge will lack the tools needed to learn from experience'.

Higher education can equip nurses with those tools, not only by giving them the opportunity to study in greater depth, but also by enabling them to make choices and to learn for themselves.

In moving towards this ideal, educational aims are shifted away from the provision of information for the student to digest. Gale (1990) suggests the job of a teacher in higher education is to liberate students' minds from prior experiences which may be limiting their potential. Intellectual and personal growth are facilitated by shifting the balance of power in this way. The teacher's task is not to proffer the requisite pieces of information to be learned, but to encourage interest and inquiry. It is more useful for students to learn to ask the right questions than for them to be taught particular answers. They need to develop the skills to seek out information for themselves, and the enthusiasm to wish to do so.

The role of the nurse teacher, within a higher education setting, is less dependent on the possession of expert knowledge, and more on the ability to facilitate learning. Teachers should feel comfortable with Gale's description of their professional duty 'to excite and stimulate students'. He points out that all learning should be enjoyable and personally rewarding, and that the task of the teacher is to create independent learners.

Facilitating learning in this way makes heavy demands on teachers, and may require a change in attitudes towards students, and towards what is learned. It may also be necessary to change the organisation of educational input. Traditionally, nurse teaching has largely consisted of conventional methods of 'chalk and talk', although there have been moves towards more student-centred learning (Burnard 1990). The timetable has tended to be full, with every session accounted for, and most entailing teacher contact. There has been little time available for reading and private study, and the teacher has been used as the main dispenser of information.

As new courses develop, it is being realised that students need time to study for themselves, time to pursue areas that interest them, and even time to waste. This creates anxiety for some teaching staff, who feel concerned that students may not be absorbing the required information. However, the aim of education should not be the acquisition of a predetermined level of knowledge, but, as Burnard and Chapman (1990) suggest, 'the development of a critical ability and the means of becoming more and more flexible and adaptable'. They argue the traditional system has not enabled recognition that there is more than one view of the world. Teachers have set the agenda for what is taught, and for what is considered to be appropriate knowledge, maintaining that there are 'truths' which it is necessary for students to learn. This does not help learners to be aware of 'knowledge as always and only tentative in nature — always subject to revision in the light of new evidence'.

The higher education environment therefore offers a more flexible framework, and should facilitate the student to set more of the programme for what is learned. It can be seen that this poses difficulties for the traditional teacher, who may feel uncomfortable with the academic approach to knowledge and research. It has been suggested (Birchenall 1991) that teachers need the skills to make use of relevant research in order to provide teaching of quality. Research awareness is high on the agenda of many courses in nursing, and most teachers promote this and incorporate it into the curriculum. However, schools of nursing have not traditionally been involved in research, and there has been little exposure to a rigorous academic climate.

The development of nursing within higher education means that both tutors and learners will have contact with those actively involved in research, and this approach should become more meaningful. Disciplines such as psychology traditionally encourage their students to act as subjects in research projects, and, by forging links with colleges of nursing, have already begun to involve student nurses in the same way. Psychology research often involves some degree of deception of its subjects, and whilst students may resent being used in this way, it certainly gives them experience from which to examine the ethics of such practices. The implementation of Project 2000 will doubtless inspire further research into areas such as the recruitment and retention of staff, and the knowledge, skills and attitudes nurses demonstrate in clinical areas. Students may well find themselves being recruited as subjects for research in the fields of nursing, education and sociology, all of which may be less hazardous than volunteering their services to psychologists.

This kind of participation heightens nurses' awareness of research, and enables them to see it as an on-going process. It also gives them invaluable experience of methodological and ethical issues, and may help them take on the role of advocate for patients involved in clinical trials. Teachers who have not had such opportunities need to recognise the learning that is occurring, and to encourage students to become involved.

It is evident that all these changes in education, such as the increased depth of study, the focus on student-orientated learning and the wider aims of such education make new demands on nurse teachers. The greater breadth of the curriculum also presents them with a challenge, by providing students with a different range of knowledge and skills. The Common Foundation Programme now gives all students exposure to courses that encourage change. Subjects such as sociology and psychology tend to increase self-awareness, and enable students to examine traditional customs and rituals. They are given courses in skills of communication and assertiveness, and encouraged to think critically. Equipped with these skills, they are beginning to question the teachers, the curriculum, the organisation and the nature of nursing itself. Again, the onus is on teachers to encourage and incite such questioning and critical attitudes, and not to feel exposed and threatened by them. Bond (1986) suggests assertiveness skills are important to help counteract the pressure of social conditioning and the 'teaching by humiliation' encountered in nursing. Teachers themselves, in some cases, are victims of this kind of education, and may need to develop their own assertiveness, as well as learning to recognise it in others as a positive attribute rather than an indication of hostility.

The academic developments engendered by Project 2000 are, then, encouraging a more assertive and critical type of student. Exposure to the social and cultural aspects of higher education will enhance this change, and will require teachers to be even more adaptable and more confident about their role. College life offers students a safe environment in which to try out new ideas, to experiment with extremes, and to develop through experience. Although the number of mature candidates is increasing, most students are young, and customarily use this time to express their changing attitudes through their dress, life-style and behaviour. Rebellion, to a degree, is sanctioned, and students can be expected to try out various modes of behaviour, before maturing to take their place in the world of work. Student politics and societies encourage intellectual stimulation, and also provide a forum for learning to argue, to be articulate and to defend a position. These are all skills of immense value to nurses in developing the profession and in acting as their patients' advocates.

Until now, nurse learners have been denied this experience, being socialised quickly into the nursing culture. They have been expected to behave as 'professionals' in the classroom (Salvage 1985), and have had the pressures and responsibilities of the clinical environment thrust upon them at an early stage of their training. Melia (1987) has described how student nurses moved between the two worlds of education and clinical practice, striving to accommodate each. Overriding importance was attached to 'fitting in' on the wards, so students quickly learnt what is acceptable behaviour in both worlds. Because of this pressure to conform, students wishing to experiment with extremes of ideas and behaviour would have had to do so covertly. Many others, lacking exposure to demonstrations of rebellion, would have missed the opportunity to try it for themselves, and thus gain in experience and maturity.

Project 2000 has at last given student nurses the chance to be students. Their supernumerary status in clinical areas reduces the pressure on them to conform, and the speed with which they have to take on responsibility. Their position within higher education promotes their chance to socialise within the environment of the students' union, as well as within the hospital. Such social change means that teachers are being presented with different patterns of behaviour by their students, which may not always seem wholly positive.

In the traditional system attendance has been obligatory, and students have been expected to conform. Teachers have seen themselves as role models, who must set standards and teach students to behave in a manner appropriate to the profession. Learners who resisted this pressure, and challenged the system, may have been among those who did not complete their training. One of the concerns addressed by the Project 2000 proposals (UKCC 1986) was that of student retention, because at that time only 65 per cent of those commencing training achieved registration. Since a large number of students withdrew from training voluntarily, the educational system must have been failing to meet their needs in some way. Orr (1990) refers to the Briggs Report (Department of Health and Social Security, 1972) which found knowledgeable students were seen by some as threatening and questions were not welcomed, and suggests such claims may still ring true today.

However, it is important to remember that the greatest pressure for the reform of nurse education has come from those who have been through the system themselves. As Naish argues in Chapter 2, despite the hidden agenda, and the pressure to conform, many nurses have emerged with their critical faculties intact, intent on improving the experience of learning for future students. This is greatly to their credit, and demonstrates the enormous strength nurses already have to look forward to change. If Project 2000 can enable those students who challenge the system to be encouraged and nurtured, instead of being coerced into conformity or lost to the profession, then this strength will be greatly reinforced. Wright (cited in McMahon and Pearson 1991) states that 'all nurses are change agents' and goes on to consider the impact a workforce of half a million would have, not only on nursing but on society in general, if all nurses were to become self-aware and knowledgeable about their influence for change. Developments in education should foster that force for change, and enable nurses to achieve their potential influence.

REVISITING ATTITUDES

In order to enhance the future impact of nursing, teachers need to look critically at their attitudes towards students, and learn to appreciate and applaud those who refuse to conform, instead of rejecting them. As links with higher education are developed, this will become an increasing challenge. The process of socialisation into college life should produce more students who are prepared to challenge and question. Some may also demonstrate attitudes which seem negative and unproductive. If experimentation with styles and ideas is sanctioned, some students will appear to go too far, and present teaching staff with modes of behaviour which appear unacceptable. Teachers have to learn that it is safe to allow students to go through this process of growth, since they will eventually achieve a greater depth of maturity. This needs to be seen as a positive demonstration of change, rather than a threat to the profession.

It can be seen that higher education presents teachers with exciting opportunities, and also with the challenge of facilitating change. The increased depth and breadth of the curriculum, the difference in educational aims, and the changing culture of the students all pose difficulties for those who have taught in the traditional system. The speed with which new courses have been developed has imposed great stress on teaching staff, and much of the focus of attention has been on the new learners. It also needs to be recognised that everybody involved in nursing is affected by these changes, both learners on other nursing courses, and clinical staff who work with these students are under particular pressure. Many have fears that existing qualifications will be devalued, and their own levels of knowledge may be undermined by higher academic standards. Whilst students adopt their new supernumerary status, clinical staff are struggling to keep the system going, and to meet both the educational demands of students and the increasing workload of the health service. If Project 2000 is to achieve its ambitions, it is vital that these tensions are acknowledged and addressed. All staff will need support through this time of change in order to develop feelings of confidence in their own value and importance, and in their active participation in change. In this way, educational innovation can be seen as belonging to nurses and building on their existing achievements, rather than as something imposed on them to replace the status quo. Thought also needs to be given to providing support and encouragement for teachers, to enable them to meet all these challenges and to help them cope with their changing role.

None of us can afford to feel complacent. We may consider ourselves already radical in our thinking and open to change. We may watch with delight as students develop their abilities to criticise and to question. However, we must all expect to face challenge, and to have to rethink our ideas. If, in education, we encourage our students to go further than we have done, we must be prepared for them to go down paths we have not even considered exploring. True education is about taking risks, about having the confidence to let go, and about empowering students to take over from us. We must learn to stand back and trust them. If we can provide a 'higher' form of education, then we can feel confident that, even if they bring the whole edifice of nursing crashing down around us, we have given these new nurses the tools to rebuild the system we have criticised for so long.

REFERENCES

Benner P (1984) *From Novice to Expert: Excellence and Power in Clinical Nursing Practice*. Menlo Park: Addison-Wesley.

Birch J A (1975) *To Nurse or not to Nurse*. London: RCN.

Birchenall P D (1991) Preparing nurse teachers for their future role. *Nurse Education Today*, **11**, 2, 100–103.

Bond M (1986) *Stress and Self-awareness: a Guide for Nurses*. Oxford: Heinemann Nursing.

Burnard P (1990) The student experience: adult learning and mentorship revisited. *Nurse Education Today*, **10**, 5, 349–54.

Burnard P and Chapman C (1990) *Nurse Education: the Way Forward*. London: Scutari Press.

Chandler J (1991) Reforming nurse education 2 — implications for teachers and students. *Nurse Education Today*, **11**, 2, 89–93.

DHSS (1972) *Report of the Commission on Nursing*. London: HMSO.

ENB (1989) *Project 2000 — A New Preparation for Practice*. London: ENB.

Gale A (1990) Applying psychology to the psychology degree. *The Psychologist: Bulletin of the British Psychological Society*, **3**, 11, 483–8.

Gott M (1983) *The Preparation of the Student for Learning in the Clinical Setting*. in Davis B D (ed) *Research into Nurse Education*. London: Croom Helm.

McMahon R and Pearson A (eds) (1991) *Nursing as Therapy*. London: Chapman and Hall.

Melia K (1987) *Learning and Working: The Occupational Socialisation of Nurses*. London: Tavistock.

Orr J G (1990) Tradition v Project 2000 — something old, something new. *Nurse Education Today*, **10**, 2, 58–62.

Robinson J (1991) Project 2000: the role of resistance in the process of professional growth. *Journal of Advanced Nursing*, **16**, 7, 820–4.

Salvage J (1985) *The Politics of Nursing*. London: Heinemann Nursing.

Skinner B F (1964) Education in 1984. *New Scientist*, **21 May**, 484.

UKCC (1986) *Project 2000: A New Preparation For Practice*. London: UKCC.

Vaughan B (1989) Two roles — one job. *Nursing Times*, **85**, 11, 52.

CHAPTER 5

Empowerment: Taking Chances, Making Changes

Charlotte Allen

'If Florence Nightingale had trained her lady pupils in assertiveness rather than obedience, perhaps nurses would be in a different place now.'
(Oakley 1984)

INTRODUCTION

This chapter celebrates the changing nature of nurse education and looks at its impact on nursing students. It explores the shift from a hierarchical, task-oriented model of training to a more humanistic, student-centred approach and the underlying principles of adult education; what this actually means for nursing students, for their tutors and for the profession of nursing. It suggests that within a student-centred approach lies the source of the empowerment of students and moreover, that the empowerment of nursing students is crucial to any development of patient-empowerment and therefore to patient-centred nursing care.

Nurses' willingness and ability to treat patients as responsible individuals with the right to make health decisions on their own behalf, depends upon the extent to which nurses themselves are valued as responsible individuals with the right to make decisions for themselves. The process which gives students the right and the responsibility to make decisions about their own learning needs lies at the heart of Project 2000.

The roots of the training that up till now have for the most part disempowered student nurses are explored, with particular regard to the relationship between nursing and medicine, the impact of gender in the organisation of nursing care and other issues related to equality of opportunity.

THE NATURE OF STUDENT-CENTRED LEARNING

Student-centred learning is often referred to, without it always being made clear what it is exactly and why it is so significant. It is a process that puts students at the centre of their own learning. The role of the tutor or mentor becomes a facilitative one, concerned with providing the resources and support which allow the student to stay in control of the learning process, a process which is unique to each individual.

Student-centred Learning	
Is about . . .	**Is not about . . .**
Raising questions	Definitive answers
Participation in	Authority over
Facilitation	Exploitation
Adult–adult relationships	Parent–child relationships
Hopes	Fears
Taking responsibility for one's own learning	Meeting other people's expectations
Challenging the status quo	Compliance
A process of learning	The completion of tasks
Realistic uncertainty	Unrealistic certainty
Education	Training
Androgogy	Pedagogy
Personal growth	A soft option!

Figure 5.1 Student-centred learning

This represents a shift of perspective of stunning dimensions: an ideological shift in the way educators perceive students, in the way students perceive themselves, and eventually in the way that the nursing profession will see nursing and the role of the nurse. The change is not only about *what* is taught, but also about *how* it is taught. The new flexible curriculum, within the framework of course requirements, goes hand in hand with a licence to explore alternative methods for achieving particular goals or outcomes, in the knowledge that different methods suit different individuals.

Such an approach treats students as adults from day one of their education. This does not remotely imply that students are expected to arrive with a prerequisite level of knowledge or expertise, but it does imply a state of mind, a belief about how people entering a professional career should be treated (Prew 1989). If students are spoonfed with facts, like Victorian schoolchildren, and coerced into keeping their heads down for three years, how can they possibly emerge from the experience as autonomous, enquiring practitioners?

Androgogy, that is the theory and practice of adult education, suggests adult education must take account of the adult's wealth of personal experience which is brought to any new learning situation, that adults need to see the relevance of the subject matter to their own learning needs, and that they need to be actively involved in the learning process (Knowles 1980). All of these elements are clearly reflected in Project 2000 course content and methodology. But if this is the Utopian picture of the new nurse education painted by the educational philosophers, it does not always feel like that to the Project 2000 student. Coping with the ambiguities of an open-ended, non-directive programme of learning presents its own special challenge. In contrast to the exercise of jumping through hoops designed by others, that characterised nurse training in the past, student-centred learning, like bottom-up management, puts much of the decision-making into the hands of the student; what to read, which avenues to explore in project work, and how to clarify one's own learning needs.

The traditional 'factory model' of nurse training (Darbyshire *et al.* 1990) with its product-oriented curriculum, produced nurses who were supposedly equipped with identical and highly standardised levels of competence and knowledge. Clearly this does nothing for the individual student's personal or professional development. What it can do is create a false sense of certainty for all those involved, when in truth the reality is never as predictable.

It should be pointed out that the move has been more gradual than might be suggested in discussions about Project 2000. Pre-registration nurse training of all types in recent years has increasingly been losing its similarity to painting-by-numbers and reflecting instead, to at least some degree, the student-centred trends attributed to Project 2000.

Facing up to the choices that students must make for themselves, coping with ambiguity, asking questions that have no straightforward answers

— what exactly should I be doing?
— where am I going on this course?
— what is this thing called nursing?
— where do I fit in?

these are the great challenges of student-centred education.

And if the reality is that there is no safety net of certainty, then a climate of learning must be cultivated, in which it is safe to feel vulnerable, to explore uncharted territory, to say 'I don't know' and to challenge the status quo. That demands new behaviours of nurse tutors, who may themselves be feeling vulnerable, and a new relationship between staff and students.

Student-centred learning is not about the tutor leaving the student to get on with it, to flounder in a *laissez-faire* pool of neglect. Far from absolving the tutor from involvement with students, it in fact makes far greater demands on the teacher (Prew 1989), creating the need for a closer tutor–student relationship, in which the tutor is responding to and nurturing each student's individual needs, rather than monitoring the successful completion of a series of tasks.

It may also imply the need for new more sensitive assessment methods (Runciman 1990), better equipped to acknowledge the *quality* as much as the quantity of learning. It may demand the courage and the commitment to loosen our attachment to 'scientism' (Johnson 1986) — that is the impulse to give the discipline of nursing academic credibility by favouring the predictable and the measurable at the expense of those aspects of the *art* of nursing, the qualitative, humanising aspects of nursing, which transcend, or at least have so far eluded, scientific quantification.

EMPOWERMENT

The relationship between student-centred learning and empowerment is an intimate one, and the success of Project 2000 may well depend upon the empowerment of nursing students. Empowerment refers to the process of taking control over one's own life decisions, placing individuals at the centre of their own unique development, in much the same way as student-centred learning does.

It is important to be clear it is not about power over others, neither is it about the abuse, exploitation or manipulation of others, nor is it about power for some (the strongest) at the expense of others (the weakest).

Its emphasis is on expanding the range of choices that people have in their own development, by reducing the constraints that are either internally imposed, for instance through ignorance, fear, lack of confidence, or externally imposed, by forces external to the self, such as other people or systems. It therefore presents opportunities and challenges very like those already discussed.

Some might dismiss the principle of self-empowerment for all as unrealistic, but it is no more unrealistic than the cherished principle of Health for All by the Year 2000 (WHO 1978). It is worth remembering there was a time when the universal vote for all adults or mass-immunisation were almost inconceivable, although as Hopson and Scally (1981) point out, self-empowerment is not an end-state so much as a process. It is not a point of arrival like a polling booth or a clinic, so much as a series of steps along a developmental path.

Apart from being central to the current direction of nurse education, self-empowerment has dramatic implications for the future direction of nursing, especially in relation to nurse–patient relationships. Figure 5.2 shows the striking parallels between student empowerment and patient empowerment.

Student-centred learning	Patient-centred care
Puts decision-making into the hands of the recipients of education, i.e. students	Puts decision-making into the hands of the recipients of health-care, i.e. patients
Individualised to suit student's needs	Individualised to suit patient's needs
Tutor's role is to support and facilitate process of learning	Nurse's role is to support and facilitate the process of recovery or coping with the lack of good health

Figure 5.2 Student empowerment and patient empowerment

The parallels are by no means coincidental. A shift of paradigm towards truly patient-centred care would have to be matched by a similar educational shift towards student-centred learning.

The relationship between the two principles is highlighted by Johnson (1986) when he states,

> 'The dysfunction of a curriculum which is not learner-centred, is that student nurses will see no relevance for patient-centred nursing, and will model the paternalism of their teachers when they plan and deliver nursing care.'

In the same vein, Burnard (1986) stresses that,

> 'If we are aiming to enable people to regain their independence, it is vital to train nurses through means that enable *them* to retain their integrity as adults.'

An analysis of the power base of the nurse–patient relationship suggests at least two compelling reasons for supporting the call for greater patient empowerment (Towl 1991): first, patients have an ethical and moral right to be central in any decisions made about them and their treatment. Second, treatment is far more likely to be effective if the patient has some control over choice of procedure and treatment, and overwhelmingly so in the case of health education, health promotion and rehabilitation.

These arguments, that of moral rightness and of increased efficacy, apply equally to the case for student empowerment. The Nursing Student's Bill of Rights (RCN 1989) echoes the sound moral principle of individual freedom and suggests a link between students' right to define their own educational needs (course requirements notwithstanding) and quality of patient care.

Research on the concept of 'locus of control' (Rotter 1966) outlines interesting differences between 'internals' (people who perceive the chief source of control over their lives to reside within themselves) and 'externals' (those who perceive control to be out of their reach or who perceive their lives to be guided by fate). Student achievement has been found to be more deeply affected by the student's own sense of powerlessness than by any objective educational variable, such as teacher qualifications, access to counselling, library resources, etc. (Coleman *et al.* 1966). This sense of powerlessness taps into issues of race, gender and social class, which will be discussed later.

A similar relationship seems to exist between internal control and health. A study of elderly patients with cancer showed the more aggressive and least docile patients tended to make a better recovery and survive longer (Canz *et al.* 1979).

Maybe nurses have something to learn from 'difficult' patients and 'difficult' students, a label often given to people who show an unwillingness to comply with other people's expectations. Moreover, people with an internal locus of control, far from displaying an exaggerated self-interest, are more likely to look outside themselves to activities which help others, and to be more committed to social and political action (presumably because they believe that their participation will make a difference).

The message for nursing is clear. The more that people, in this case students, feel they do have some power to influence what happens to them, the more likely they are to use that influence for the benefit of others and the nursing profession.

If self-empowerment serves to benefit both self, others and the community, what then are its attributes? Figure 5.3 offers an operational definition of self-empowerment.

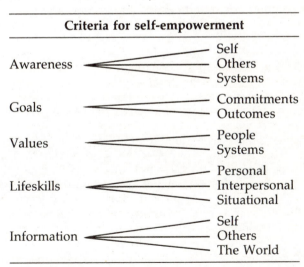

Taken and slightly adapted from *Lifeskills Teaching*, Hopson and Scally (1981)

Figure 5.3 An operational definition of self-empowerment

Awareness of self, others and society is well rooted in the inter-personal skills component of the Common Foundation Programme. Implicit in the development of self-awareness is a sense of one's own worth and uniqueness. It is an awareness of others that puts caring at the core of the new curriculum, not because nurses have not cared enough in the past, on the contrary, because they have seriously undervalued their own caring qualities, qualities like empathy and understanding that lie at the heart of nursing excellence. Awareness of the wider social, political and environmental issues that affect health are also needed if self-empowerment is to give rise to effective action.

Goals are not in themselves evidence of self-empowerment behaviour. But if self-empowerment is about believing change is best brought about by informed choice, rather than by coercion (Tones *et al.* 1991), then one needs to be clear about what the desired change might look like. For goals to be indicators of self-empowerment, they must be specific in terms of outcome, and they must be 'owned' by those who set them. That is to say, the goal-setter must believe in their value and be committed to their attainment. Goals imposed by others, or the result of internal 'scripts' (Steiner 1974), that is internalised messages usually of a judgemental kind, which dictate the way in which a person behaves as a result of early conditioning, are de-powering rather than empowering.

If self-empowerment is to be for all people, not just the privileged few, then certain *values* are implicit (Anderson 1986). Respect for the intrinsic worth of all people regardless of age, gender, race, ability or any other human variable, clearly lies at the very heart of any philosophy of self-empowerment for all. To respect others presupposes a healthy respect for oneself. Selflessness may have a place in nursing, but beware the 'compulsive carer'. The 'compulsive carer' puts a low value on taking good care of herself. Her (and it is often a female) low self-esteem means that looking after others becomes a way, maybe the only way, of justifying her own worth. This disempowered behaviour demands that the patient or client be disempowered as well, in order that the carer can feel really needed. Such a spiral of disempowered dependency does no favours for anyone.

True self-empowerment also means actions are consistent with values. Or as a wise university tutor once advised me, 'If you want to know where a person's, an organisation's or even a government's values really lie, look not at what they want to tell you, but at what they actually do.'

Lifeskills cover the gamut of behavioural skills that increase the range of alternatives open to a person; from personal skills like learning to manage one's own stress, to interpersonal skills such as listening to the real meaning behind another person's words, to situational skills such as how to get the best out of the college library, or to lobby for educational change.

Paradoxically, for a service dedicated to caring for other people, the business of caring for each other as health care professionals is still one of the most seriously undervalued, and consequently under-developed, lifeskills in the Health Service.

The link between staff morale and patient recovery has been clearly demonstrated and research shows most stress in the NHS is due to a lack of perceived support and the sense of 'teamlessness' that follows (Hiscox 1991). Perhaps surprisingly, in a time of organisational uncertainty and professional insecurity, it seems that the demands of the job are in fact less critical in perceiving and coping with stress, than access to an adequate level of ongoing support.

Yet it is only very recently that we, as a profession, have started inching our way towards the development of staff support systems which could harness some of the interpersonal skills that nurses use in their interactions with patients, and use them in their professional relationships with each other.

Hiscox's (1991) personal experience of setting up a staff support group showed that nurses valued holding meetings before and not as a consequence of a crisis. The empowered person pre-empts the crisis where possible by taking action beforehand. This requires not only foresight and planning, however, but more importantly the recognition that support networks or systems, both formal and informal, are a fundamental prerequisite to good health and not simply a strategy for coping with crisis.

The importance of *information*, the last of Hopson's component's of self-empowerment, cannot be over-estimated. A person without information is a person without power and the most tyrannical of regimes knows this well. To withhold information is a potent form of disempowerment. A college of nursing's attitude towards information therefore, is a significant measure of its commitment to the creation of a genuinely empowering environment.

Developing the self-empowering skills associated with access to information would include straightforward retrieval skills, in a library for example, learning how to gain access to those people who hold relevant information, the willingness on their part to share it, and the skilful evaluation and use of information to enhance any subsequent decision-making process.

ADVOCACY AND WHISTLEBLOWING

No discussion of self-empowerment for students would be complete without mentioning the business of advocacy and whistle-blowing. The relationship between the empowerment of oneself and the ability to advocate for others is a powerful one. Learning to speak up for oneself and one's peers is crucial, and from this arises the courage and the capacity to advocate for one's patients. For if nurses do not speak up for the vulnerable people that they care for, who else will?

The skills and inclination for patient advocacy cannot be taken for granted. They need to have a central place in the educational curriculum and be given the same priority as all other aspects of good patient care.

Students need the opportunity to explore these issues and their implications for nursing practice in the safety of a classroom environment, before practising them in clinical placements; a classroom environment in which it is safe to admit to feeling afraid, to make mistakes, to bring back experience from clinical placements for discussion, and to know that tutors will listen with unswerving support (Allen 1991).

THE 'VICTIM' CONSCIOUSNESS OF THE NURSING CULTURE AND ITS HISTORICAL ROOTS

One indication of the growing empowerment of the nursing profession shows nurses moving out of the shadow of the medical model of *cure*, dominated by doctors, and staking a claim to an autonomous body of knowledge and expertise that broadly defines nursing as a culture of *care*.

The fact that this has not always been the case is explained by the historical roots of medicine and nursing and the role of gender traditionally reflected in nurse–doctor relationships. Many writers have highlighted the parallels between these relationships and the

Victorian family (Salvage 1985; Oakley 1984; Robinson 1991). For doctor read father; the patriarch and head of the household (even when absent), to whom all the most significant decisions are referred. Witness how often this is still true, especially in a hospital sub-culture, even when the decision falls within the domain of nursing expertise, such as how best to care for a wound, or where the territory is indisputably 'female', such as on a labour ward.

For mother, read nurse, ward sister or even matron; the matriarchal head of household duties, who keeps all household staff under strict supervision (hence the popular image of the strict ward sister as a 'dragon'). In the 19th Century, experience as a domestic servant was the only qualification required for nursing, and a preoccupation with damp-dusting, pillow-case openings facing away from the door and the rigours of the sluice are still within the living memory of many nurses.

In this nuclear-family model of nursing care, the patient is of course the child. Father and mother (doctor and nurse) take care of and make judgements about the welfare of their children (patients).

A model of nurse training based on these guidelines places the student firmly in the role of the child. Once again the parallels between the student and the patient are clear. And just as legislation last century took children from the factories and into the classroom, so recently has legislation stopped student nurses being exploited as under-paid and under-valued workers and placed their learning squarely in an educational context.

The vast majority of people working in health care all over the world are women, both in the developing and the industrialised world, with the exception of the medical profession which is male-dominated. Even where this is not numerically the case (as in Britain, where the gender split is 50:50, amongst doctors qualifying), the tendency is for men to monopolise the most senior positions. This is true even where women become doctors and men become nurses. In a nursing profession composed of 90 per cent women, 50 per cent of its most senior managers and educationalists are men (Hardie 1987).

The question is, why do men hold a disproportionate share of senior nursing positions? Oakley (1984) suggests the disparity is one of assertiveness; that women in general, and nurses and midwives in particular, need assertiveness training. She also claims Florence Nightingale never challenged this link between nursing and womanhood, when she tried to professionalise nurses, and that nursing is disempowered by a notion of womanhood which values the submissive qualities of women and subtly punishes women who display assertiveness by labelling them 'aggressive' or 'unfeminine'.

This picture of docility does have another side to it however. Altruism (that is the ability to care and the tendency to put other people's needs before one's own) is commonly perceived as a 'female' quality. The centrality of caring lies at the heart of most definitions of good nursing and emerges clearly as the nursing attribute most valued by patients. It is this capacity to care that is both the greatest strength and the greatest vulnerability of the profession. A strength because altruism is recognised and valued as a social strength, but a vulnerability because it is often played out at great personal cost to the nurse. If it is taken seriously as a strength, where do we see altruism applauded? Certainly it has never won fame or fortune, and the altruistic person is not even meant to seek such plaudits. In a culture where money and status denote the worth of a person's work, it is difficult to see exactly how the value of altruism is heralded.

In the same way, it is sometimes difficult to remember that the complex and challenging skills of fundamental nursing care, such as bathing the immobilised elderly person, or just being with a person in unbearable physical pain or emotional anguish, sometimes described as 'high-touch' nursing, are at least as important and valuable as 'high-tech' nursing, with all its connotations of medical glamour and technical trail-blazing.

It is this disparity between 'doing good and feeling bad' (Oakley 1984) that undermines nurses' confidence in their caring work and feeds the image of the nurse as victim or martyr or 'angel' even. The temptation is for nurses to find affirmation through virtue, if they do not find affirmation through achievement.

This is confirmed by Miller's work (1977) on the personality characteristics associated with people belonging to subordinate and dominant social groups. People who belong to subordinate groups, whether children, black or minority ethnic people, women or nurses, tend to be socialised into patterns of behaviour which induce dependency, passivity and thinking about other people's welfare. People in dominant social groups, on the other hand, adults, white people, men, doctors, are more likely to develop qualities of independence, initiative and putting their own welfare before other people's (Oakley 1984).

Is it therefore going to take an influx of male nursing students for nursing to lose its subordinate status? And if this is the case where does it leave nursing? Where does it leave women in nursing? And who exactly will be the beneficiaries of such a move? Clearly issues of equal opportunities in nursing are as pertinent as ever.

EQUAL OPPORTUNITIES

It is sobering to discover that in a profession numerically dominated by women the challenge of equal opportunities for all nurses has not yet been remotely met.

One of the original aims of Project 2000 was to respond to the dwindling pool of young, white, female school-leavers that nursing had hitherto tapped into, and attract instead, a more varied range of potential recruits.

Clearly, disparity of opportunity according to gender in nursing is as prevalent as ever. Not only do men in nursing rise to the most senior positions more quickly and in disproportionate numbers, an issue examined in detail by Dolan in Chapter 5, but there exists painfully scant acknowledgement of the special needs of student mothers or fathers, and most especially single parents. Apart from a handful of courses specifically designed to meet the domestic needs of student parents, Project 2000 has so far failed to acknowledge that students with children are a valuable resource for nursing and need robust, demonstrable support.

It is an assumption based on ageism that organises nurse education to suit young, child-free adults with no demanding family commitments. Nursing students in their 30's, 40's or 50's are far more likely to be carers in their domestic lives, caring either for children or older relatives.

As for encouraging a student population that even remotely reflects the diverse ethnic profile of the multi-cultural population that nurses serve, we have scarcely begun to address the issue. Many nurses would be shocked and upset to be accused of racism and would counter the accusation with evidence of their good nursing practice in minority ethnic communities. Institutionalised racism, as it exists in the health service, is not the crude expression of anti-black feeling. It is the pernicious and subtle marginalisation of people from minority ethnic groups, which takes for granted that black health care workers are found in disproportionate numbers in the lowest paid and least skilled jobs (nursing auxiliaries and health care assistants for example). It is a marginalisation that forgets even to ask why there are so few black ward sisters and charge nurses and where the black managers are. In educational terms, it is a marginalisation that slips 'race and ethnicity' into the curriculum as an item that can seemingly be wrapped up and parcelled away in one or two sessions. (Far better this than nothing at all, however.)

How far does current nurse education, including Project 2000, meet the needs of students from black and minority ethnic groups? Does it even recognise they may have special academic and personal needs?

Any method of assessment which depends upon writing good English at speed (in a timed examination, for example), discriminates against those for whom English is a second language. And yet often these are the very people who bring with them a maturity and a breadth of perspective, born of straddling more than one culture, that the profession badly needs. They are far too precious to lose simply because they have failed to meet the ethnocentric standards of a dominant white group which has not recognised their own particular strengths.

THE USE OF LANGUAGE

Educational psychologists are still debating whether language precedes thought or thought precedes language. Either way it has a powerful effect on the way in which people perceive reality. Language conveys a lot about where the power resides in a team, an organisation or a culture and can be used to empower or disempower. It is used with chilling effect to reinforce the inequalities just discussed.

Midwifery tutors still make generic reference to 'pink' babies, and the language of sexism is rife throughout the health service. Tutors refer to 'models of man' when 'models of the person' is a far more acceptable and accurate alternative. Using the word 'chairman' or 'spokesman' as if they were generic terms, perpetuates the myth that the person taking the chair or speaking on behalf of others is more likely to be male than female (Platzer and Rawlings-Anderson 1991).

Project 2000 will be doing nursing the greatest service if it is vigilant in its use of non-oppressive language. By the same token, it is not nit-picking to insist that pre-registration diploma and undergraduate students are called *nursing students* rather than *student nurses*. First and foremost, they are students, like all other higher education students, with three years to explore and study and grow. Student nurses on the other hand, do their training within a context of service provision, because they are in essence employed 'apprentice' nurses. To call these students 'traditional', as if the training they are currently receiving is already out-of-date, is not helpful, even if a widely acceptable alternative has not so far been coined. Perhaps it is time to call *all* students of nursing, 'nursing students'.

THE STRENGTH OF THE COMMON FOUNDATION PROGRAMME AS A SOURCE OF EMPOWERING IDEAS

One of Project 2000's great strengths is the exposure it offers all students during the Common Foundation Programme, to all branches of the profession. This presents the opportunity for students to be influenced by the span of some of the most radical, empowering and innovative thinking in current nursing practice, ideas such as:

— the *demedicalisation* of normal childbirth in maternity services,
— the *real inclusion of the entire family* when nursing the sick child (why not elsewhere as well?)
— the *multi-disciplinary nature* of community care,
— the models of *client-empowerment* emerging from current thinking on health promotion,
— the injunction to aim for Health for All by the Year 2000 (WHO) and the acknowledgement of *global health needs* within a context of environmental health,
— the notion of *normalisation* in caring for people with severe physical and learning difficulties, and
— the *humanistic, psychotherapeutic perspective* of much mental health nursing.

These ideas are often not as prevalent in the dominant culture of adult general nursing (especially where care is hospital-based). Adult general nursing is still dogged by its military heritage, which pre-dates its subservient role in the medical model of cure. Notice the predilection for belts, buckles, stripes and other military paraphernalia to denote rank amongst hospital nurses (Salvage 1985). Notice also the pervasiveness of militaristic language; charge nurse, auxiliary, theatre (as in theatre of war?), and now even 'cohort' to describe an intake of Project 2000 students.

The challenge for mental health and learning disabilities nursing on the other hand, has been to free itself of the shackles of its own historical beginnings in the lunatic asylum (*sic*) and the work-house, with all the associated connotations of shame, disrepute and second class citizenship.

So if nursing looks to its 'minority' branches for some of its most innovative and inspiring ideas, it is ironic that so many of these ideas and the ones that return power firmly to the client, should fall within what are often the most under-resourced (and therefore the most under-valued?) services, the areas of nursing which depend upon high-touch rather than high-tech nursing.

CONCLUSION

Project 2000 is an act of faith for the nursing profession. It has engaged everyone involved with nurse education (including clinical practitioners) in a stunningly different process of pre-registration training, and no-one yet knows exactly what the result will be. In contrast to the authoritarianism and bureaucracy of previous training, which enslaved rather than empowered student nurses, Project 2000 is designed to foster creativity, flexibility and autonomy.

In spite of the academic foundations of diplomate and graduate nurse education, Project 2000 is at least as much about the *art* of nursing — the primacy of caring — as about the *science* of nursing. As Darbyshire *et al.* (1990) say,

> 'In an era of health care dominated by high technology, commercialism and service cuts, people are now even more reliant on nurse caring that recognises their humanity and individuality and responds in ways which connect and confirm rather than mechanise and alienate.'

Student-centred learning has striking parallels with patient-centred care. If the profession truly believes in a process of nursing that enables people to regain their independence, then it is vital that nurse education allows students to retain their integrity as adults (Burnard 1986).

The new curriculum will better prepare nurses to function effectively in the arena of social and political issues, and can be expected to develop not only decision-making skills but also policy-making skills (Tierney 1990). But of course, ultimately its success will depend upon the entire nursing profession and its willingness to embrace the new and challenging values inherent in Project 2000 principles. It does not and should not set Project 2000 students apart from other students and nurses. Its success depends upon all students and all nurses jumping on board and moving forward together. If it is owned and valued by all nurses, it will place nurses and their patients at the very centre of health care, empowered by their ability to make informed and sensitive choices.

And there will be much to celebrate . . .

REFERENCES

Allen C (1991) A profession caring. *Nursing Standard,* **5**, 51, 45–6.

Anderson J (1986) Health skills: the power to choose. *Health Education Journal,* **45**, 1, 19–24.

Burnard P (1986) Encountering adults. *Senior Nurse,* **4**, 4, 30–1.

Canz P *et al.* (1979) The psycho-social impact of cancer on the elderly: a comparison with younger patients. *Journal of the American Geriatric Society,* **33**, 429–435.

Coleman J S *et al.* (1966) Equality of Educational Opportunity *Report from Office of Education. US Government Printing Office,* Washington D.C.

Darbyshire P, Steward B, Jamieson L and Tongue C (1990) New Domains in Nursing. *Nursing Times,* **86**, 27, 73–5.

Hardie L (1987) The male model. *Nursing Times,* **83**, 21, 36–8.

Hiscox C (1991) Stress and its management. *Nursing Standard,* **5**, 21, 36–40.

Hopson B and Scally M (1981) *Lifeskills Teaching* London: McGraw-Hill (UK).

Johnson M (1986) A message for the teacher. *Nursing Times,* **82**, 54, 41–3.

Knowles M (1980) *The Modern Practice of Adult Education* (2nd edition). Chicago: Follet.

Miller J B (1977) *Towards a New Psychology of Women* Boston: Beacon Press.

Oakley A (1984) The importance of being a nurse. *Nursing Times,* **80**, 50, 24–7.

Platzer H and Rawlings-Anderson K (1991) Sexist language — why fuss? *Nursing Standard,* **5**, 22, 54–6.

Prew C (1989) Thoughts on a new curriculum. *Nursing Times,* **85**, 10, 70–1.

Robinson J (1991) Educational conditioning. *Nursing Times,* **87**, 10, 28–31.

Rotter J B (1966) Generalised expectancies for internal versus external control of reinforcement. *Psychological monographs* 80:1, entire issue.

RCN (1989) *Nursing Students' Bill of Rights* (2nd edition). London: RCN.

Runciman P (1990) *Competence-Based Education and the Assessment and Accreditation of Work-Based Learning in the Context of Project 2000 Programmes of Nurse Education: A Literature Review*. Edinburgh: Scottish National Board for Nursing, Midwifery and Health Visiting.

Salvage J (1985) *The Politics of Nursing*. London: Heinemann Nursing.

Steiner C (1974) *Scripts people live*. New York: Grove Press.

Tierney R (1990) Strategies for empowerment. *Nursing Standard*, **4**, 47, 32–4.

Tones K, Tilford S and Robinson Y (1991) *Health Education: Effectiveness and Efficiency*. London: Chapman Hall.

Towl G (1991) Scrutinising the power complex. *Nursing Standard*, **5**, 50, 45–6.

WHO (1978) *Health for All by the Year 2000; Declaration of Alma-Ata*. Geneva: WHO.

CHAPTER 6

Gender and Change

Brian Dolan

'Men have always been a touchy subject in nursing.' (Gaze 1987)

INTRODUCTION

Men in nursing occupy an anomalous position. They are a statistical minority in a predominantly female profession, forming approximately 9 per cent of the total nursing workforce, yet fill a disproportionately high percentage of senior posts.

This chapter will examine some of the reasons for this apparent inequality and what Project 2000 may achieve in rectifying it. First, men's development in nursing will be explored from a historical perspective before considering their current position in the nursing world and its meaning. Finally, a view will be offered of the future of men in nursing, based on educational and attitudinal changes both within and outwith the nursing profession. The educational change that is Project 2000 could be the catalyst for a change that will lead to greater equality for both men and women in nursing.

A HISTORICAL REVIEW

When teaching the history of our profession to students of nursing much time is spent waxing lyrical on the undoubted contribution of Florence Nightingale, who did much to legitimise nursing as a profession. However widespread this view, it undermines the part that men have played historically. Although nursing today can be clearly recognised as being predominantly female, there have been times, suggests Jones (1984), when men have been far more involved in nursing care.

Some of the earliest historical evidence of men's role in nursing exists with the brotherhood of Parabaloni in the 3rd Century and the St Basil's Monks who were performing nursing duties in the 6th Century (McAllen 1961). During the Crusades, in the medieval times, members of the male military orders could be found functioning as nurses and hospital administrators (Hase 1977).

Orders such as the Hospitallers of St John of Jerusalem and the Teutonic Knights were also founded at this time to ensure a supply of soldiers fit for battle. Bush (1976) proposes that men looked after the sick because women were believed to be too fragile to carry out this work. Jones (1984) also believes the concept of nursing and the need for nursing care was perhaps very different from the aims of nursing today. While the medieval nurse's aim was to return wounded soldiers to the fighting fray, nurses today are concerned with returning patients and clients to optimum functional ability (Henderson 1966).

The passage of several centuries has obliterated the memory of these medieval 'nurses'. As time went by, women increasingly took over this role, initially for structural economic reasons. There were few men left after the wars to farm the land and gradually they began to abdicate the responsibility of looking after the sick to women. The efforts of the men was now concentrated on ensuring that enough food was available to nourish the community. Indeed, the word 'nursing' is itself Latinate, meaning 'to nourish'. Later, women were deemed more suitable than men to nurse as values such as 'caring' and 'nurturing', became increasingly seen as 'feminine' instincts.

But if nursing was born, through the religious orders, in the Church, then it was bred in the army. By the middle of the 19th Century nursing was developing as a quasi-religious, quasi-military occupation and men were distinctly discouraged from joining.

Dingwall (1972) states this was because

> 'nursing was developing as a reflection of Victorian middle-class family life, with the father figure of the doctor symbolising patriarchal authority over all members and the matron exercising matriarchal control over women and women's work'.

Men as nurses did not feature in this scenario. Dingwall (1972) proposes that men were excluded both by the creation of a public image of nursing as an exclusively female occupation and by discriminatory recruitment policies, particularly in the elite fields of general nursing and midwifery. The exception to this was in psychiatry and in learning disabilities nursing. Here, men were employed in 'lunatic asylums' (*sic*) as custodians rather than nurses and these areas of care did not develop as specialities until much later.

In viewing nursing as an occupation for upper-middle-class women, providing both a training for marriage and a respectable status for those unable to marry, it also began, argues Darbyshire (1986), to delineate and emphasise the 'different' concepts of caring and curing. Doctors — the curers — were exclusively men, and seen as dynamic, scientific and requiring a high degree of intelligence. On the other hand, nurses — the carers — were almost exclusively women, and were seen practical and on a more pedestrian academic footing.

The issue of gender also ranks highly in explaining the position of nurses and their situation within nursing. The nurse was seen as remarkably similar in character to the 'good woman', argues McKay (1989). Generations of nursing students were trained in a tradition that assumed

> 'she (the student) will never make a good nurse unless she regards her time as the hospital's and not her own'. (*Lancet* Commission on Nursing 1932)

The perception that nurses are born not made was still evident in Department of Health campaigns right up to the early 1980's. It also subliminally suggested that unless you were prepared to make sacrifices (in all senses of the word) you would not make it as a nurse.

Despite the real social and employment discrimination faced by men wishing to enter nursing, by 1901, some 5700 men were members of the profession (Boorer 1968). However, in 1919, when the register of nurses was established, men were relegated to having their name on a separate list and remained there for the next 30 years. By 1931, the total number of men in nursing had reached 15 000. In 1950, five years after the Second World War, there were 1719 male registered nurses in general nursing, nearly six times the pre-war figure (Browne and Stones 1973).

While by now there were a total of 25 600 trained and untrained men in nursing, constituting 17 per cent of the total nursing workforce, the war had also codified civilian discrimination against men. Female nurses, including many untrained auxiliary nurses, were automatically given officer status in the Queen Alexandra Imperial Nursing Services (QA's) whilst men in the Royal Army Medical Corps (RAMC) remained in the ranks.

At this stage in the modern history of nursing, any inequalities appear to have been one way and men had limited opportunity to influence change in nursing. Even the Royal College of Nursing (RCN) would not allow men to become members until 1960. It is perhaps a measure of the influence men have gained in nursing in the last three decades that by 1982 Trevor Clay became the RCN's General Secretary.

GENDER AND SEXUALITY

Jones (op. cit.) suggests:

> 'Nursing grew at a time when women were finding their feet and preparing themselves for competition in a male dominated society.' (p. 6)

Excluding men from nursing ensured a female dominance in one of the very few areas open to 'respectable' women. Nursing offered the newly franchised woman an alternative (Hass 1977).

Marx (1867), however, had an opposing view, arguing that women were in fact a reserve army of labour, useful in crises such as wars, but expected to return to the home and hearth when the need for them had passed. Nursing was useful in keeping women in readiness without threatening the male domain.

But the men who wanted to enter this domain could not have been 'real' men, so therefore must be homosexual. The rationale for this, suggests Webb (1985), goes as follows; men who enter nursing couldn't make it in a man's world thus have only a woman's world open to them. In nursing, the attributes of gentility, compassion and caring are encouraged, but are seen as feminine rather than masculine characteristics. The men in nursing are also, initially at least, subordinate to women. Hence, if their masculinity is in question, then it is not such a conceptual leap to begin to question their sexual orientation.

There is no evidence to support this hypothesis or the belief that there is a greater preponderance of homosexual men in nursing, although Littlewood (1991) suggests that the heterosexual man in nursing is continually expected to justify his sexual interests without compromising his 'feminine' task. Equally, Salvage (1985) proposes that if there are more gay men in nursing it could be because

> 'it does not seem to demand the macho atrributes of stereotypical masculinity'.

One may take this argument a stage further when offering reasons why so many men enter senior nursing and management posts, that is, the reassertion of masculinity. If society views men who enter nursing as not real men, then arguably they could then be perceived as 'pseudo-women'. This threatens men's role in our patriarchal society, hence another (perhaps subconscious) motive for entering the dynamic 'masculine' fields of management and education. Sexuality should not matter in nursing, but the truth is it does, and a lot of emotional and professional energy is expended exploring its impact, perhaps to the occasional detriment of the other, equally important issues facing the profession, not least Project 2000.

Perhaps on a more pragmatic level, although this is now changing, nursing has traditionally been poorly paid. This may have had as much to do with the perceived value of women in society as the financial importance of the role. Men, also traditionally, have been viewed as the main breadwinners in the family and through financial and social pressures it became incumbent on them to enter the more senior, better paid posts, even when they might have preferred to stay by the bedside.

As a consequence, nursing is no longer a female but a male dominated profession — that is male doctors, male nurse managers operating within a patriarchal society. In the three decades that men have had the most influence in nursing it has undergone a masculinisation. Nurses are now far more involved in the curative aspects of nursing once the reserve of doctors (read men). High-tech areas of care, such as accident and emergency and intensive care units, have greater status in nursing than the high-touch areas such as elderly care, mental health, or community nursing.

This is despite the fact, particularly in relation to the education of Project 2000 students, that they are areas of care that have much

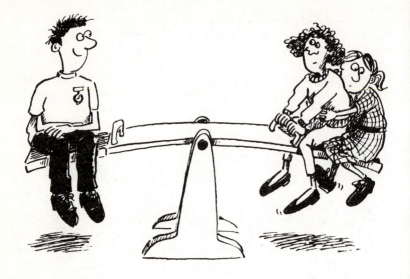

to offer in the form of innovative practices such as complementary therapies, primary nursing and nursing development units. It begs the rhetorical question whether the highly successful *Jimmys*, *Hospital Watch* or *Casualty* television series would have lasted so long had they been set in a community home for those with learning disabilities.

Too often it seems, the curative, high-profile aspects of the nurse's role has been at the expense of the subtler but no less important caring elements of what nurses do. The art of nursing is in danger of being sacrificed on a scientific altar. All too frequently we delegate 'tasks' such as bed-bathing to students or ancillary staff and describe them as 'basic' (read feminine) nursing care. As Moccia (1988) points out, nursing has the charge of caring in a society that devalues such activities.

If the reasons why this belief has come about are complex, a significant factor must be the gender divisions of our society which laid the foundation for reports such as Salmon (Ministry of Health 1966). It was an examination of the nursing management structure and may be best known outside nursing in calling for, and seeing the demise of the title 'matron'. Its authors were openly critical of female authority and management and it set the scene for an explosion in the number of men going into nurse education and management posts. Choon and Skevington (1992) note:

> 'In 1971, on average there were seven women for every man in post. However, looking at senior posts of chief and principal nursing officer and charge nurse, the proportion of women to men was only three to one.' (p. 90)

In a critique of the report, Carpenter (1977) writes of the Salmon Report's (op. cit.) implicit sexism. For instance, one reads of Salmon's complaints that once women are moved from being ward nurses to adminstrators 'they seem unable to make decisions'.

The solution was clear. Female nurses might be good at direct, hands-on patient care, but for middle and senior management posts more tough minded, dynamic, rational qualities were required. It was no accident that these were the qualities that were traditionally assumed to be within men's domain. Men could, and did, move into a more male-friendly nursing management and education structure (Gaze 1987).

It is also striking that they could operate according to an industrial model of professionalised management and an organisational structure which takes the form of bureaucratic management more than a collegial model of professional behaviour. The 'female' professions have not developed simply as professions parallel to those of men, for men have now entered them and re-established themselves at the top of the hierarchy (Goody 1982).

So, just how successful have men been and equally important what sort of men are they? Some of the answers to this question can be found in a study by Hardy (1987). She found as well as being disproportionately successful (Figure 6.1), they also have significantly different characteristics to their female counterparts (Figure 6.2).

While this study occurred before the introduction of clinical grading, which is meant to reward nurses for staying at the bedside, the men in Hardy's work were shown to move more quickly through the ranks than women, taking 8.4 years to reach their first nursing officer post, compared to women who took 14.5 years. Their career also tended to be more vertical than the lateral career directions of the women in the study, who tended to gather certificates. This is borne out by the fact that these women had on average five qualifications compared to the men's 3.5. Dingwall and MacIntosh (1978) describe this as the 'certificate gatherer syndrome'.

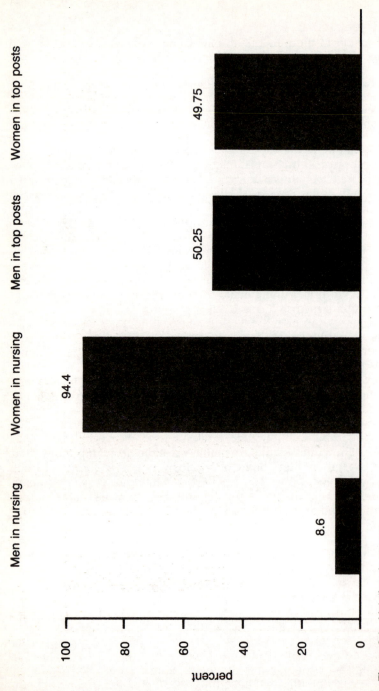

Figure 6.1 Male/female nurses

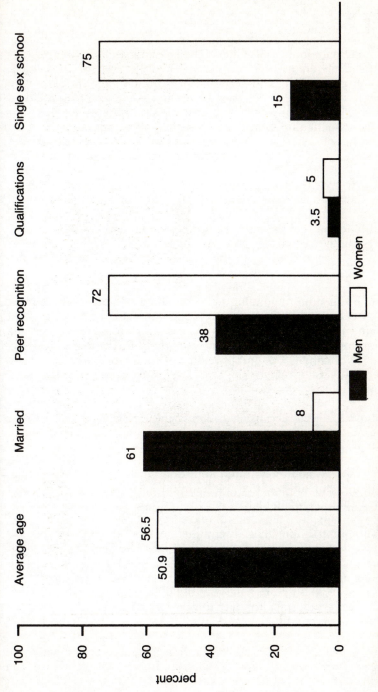

Figure 6.2 Characteristics of male/female nurses senior managers

One of the most fascinating aspects of Hardy's (op. cit.) study is the difference in marital status of the two groups. Sixty-one per cent of the men were married compared to just 8 per cent of the women. Two issues are revealed here. First, whilst marriage should not be seen as a measure of heterosexuality, it does discredit the 'all men nursing are homosexual' hypothesis. It also appears, on the basis of the evidence offered, to suggest that for women to succeed in nursing, marriage is not compatible with a career and greater personal sacrifices were (and are?) frequently required. It is also more common for men to move with their whole families than it is for women to do the same, suggesting once more that careers are perceived as somehow more important for men than women.

Hardy found that the men studied appeared to 'break all the rules' by going to the 'wrong' primary and secondary schools, not being middle class and going to the 'wrong' nursing schools. This did not, it can be seen, prevent them from succeeding.

But, if the men in nursing had one singular advantage, it must have been in having a mentor. The value to the individual of having a mentor cannot be overstated and Project 2000 students stand to gain from having mentors early in their careers. Authors such as Sheehy (1976) and Levison (1978 cited in Hardy 1987) state mentor–protégé relationships are critical to career development. Hardy defines a mentor as

> 'someone who successfully assists younger individuals to meet their career goals through modelling, advising, teaching, guiding and/or promoting'.

An effective mentor is often someone who holds a senior position and can offer advice and support based on experience and understanding of the situation.

Given all this positive discrimination one should not be too surprised that by the end of the 1980's, the UK Central Council for Nurses, Midwives and Health Visitors (UKCC), the Royal College of Nursing (RCN), the Confederation of Health Service Employees (COHSE) and the National Union of Public Employees (NUPE) had male leaders despite the fact that 90 per cent of their registrees/ members were women.

It is the apparent inequality of this situation that once more begs a rhetorical question. Given the dominance of men in this profession, what difference can Project 2000 make? The final part of this chapter will examine how, through educational and attitudinal changes, these imbalances may be rectified in a way that will not just affect our profession but our society as a whole.

NURSES AS AGENTS OF SOCIAL CHANGE IN THE ERADICATION OF INEQUALITY

The National Health Service (NHS) is one of the largest employers in the world with over one million employees. Approximately 500 000 of these are nurses, 90 per cent of whom are women. But while entrepreneurial, market-driven forces are being introduced into the NHS to develop a business of health, others such as the Royal College of Nursing (1989) have argued that the changes brought about by the NHS Act 1990 addressed the wrong agenda for health and thus did not truly reflect the needs of an ageing, more chronically ill society. While more women than men use the Health Service, it is predominantly men who make the decisions that affect peoples lives.

Unions themselves have not been above fault in the past, as Osborne (1989) found, with the Trades Union Congress (TUC) in 1947 stating 'the most important place for a woman is in the home'.

The conservatism of nursing has often served to reinforce this view with the widespread belief that nursing is good preparation for motherhood and home-making (Kalisch and Kalisch 1982). Yet if there is a future for equality in nursing it is, as in so many other things, in social change through education.

The concept of social change, argues Akinsanya (1989), is one of the most important aspects in any society and is inevitable. Nursing, he continues,

> 'can be viewed as a potential for social change both in terms of its statutory provisions and the professional socialization of those who practise it'.

First, however, it is necessary to understand the forces of change. Evolution effects change at a pace that cannot always be identified and is accomplished with minimum disruption to existing practices. An example of this within the context of men in nursing was their ineligibility to join the RCN for the first 44 years of its existence. At the opposite extreme, revolution is change which occurs so rapidly that it causes great discomfort. It is also difficult to ascertain which direction the changes will take. There are no clear-cut examples of revolution that can be directly related to nursing, although it could be argued that the length of time it has taken Project 2000 to come into being means that describing it as a revolution in the way nurses are educated is not a definition that stands up to scrutiny!

A more accurate way of describing both the educational changes of Project 2000 and the third type of social change is reform. Reform is legitimised by a process in which the nature of existing social conditions is generally considered inappropriate, obsolete, irrelevant or simply ripe for change. It is the process that led us to Project 2000 and it is a process that could lead men and women in nursing to compete on a more equal footing.

Implicit in the philosophy of Project 2000 is the education of nurses who will become independent, autonomous practitioners of care. Elsewhere (Dolan 1990; Wright 1991) it has been suggested that if nurses (read women) are self-aware, autonomous, skilled change agents, then the implications not just for nursing and nurses but for society as a whole are profound. Remembering that over 90 per cent of Britain's 500 000 nurses are women, the ripple effect could be felt throughout. Nursing could also become a catalyst for real change in how women and their role in society are seen.

For Project 2000 to meet these objectives it is vital that a change of attitude occurs within nursing. Project 2000 nurses will only be as self-aware and autonomous as the profession lets them. An examination of the profession's own prejudices and fears is needed so it may move forward from its current adolescent traumas towards a maturity that is not always self-evident.

Part of that challenge lies in valuing clinical practice as the *raison d'être* for nursing rather than seeing this role as a predominantly female one (Marrow 1990). Nursing may quite simply be a practice, but its practice is far from simple (Pearson 1992). This offers a challenge that will stimulate and exercise nurses, irrespective of their sex.

In conclusion, the reader could well be forgiven for assuming the writer believes that men should not be nurses if they are inclined to use their nursing qualifications as a mere stepping stone into management or education, and in any case, men make poor nurses. On the contrary, writing both as a man and a nurse, the writer does not accept the anatomy-is-destiny argument.

There are good nurses and there are bad nurses. Their sex is incidental.

What is not incidental, however, is the fact that men have fared far better in nursing than their numbers would suggest. Equality is not about positive discrimination in favour of one or other group, but about all groups competing *equally*. Project 2000 offers the opportunity to make that happen.

Time will tell whether or not it succeeds.

REFERENCES

Akansanya J (1989) Nursing: an agent for social change. (Unpublished)

Boorer D (1968) Men nurses in Britain. *Nursing Outlook*, **16**, 11, 24–26.

Brown R G S and Stones R W H (1973) *The Male Nurse*. Birkenhead: Williams Brothers.

Bush P (1976) The male nurse: a challenge to traditional role identities. *Nursing Forum*, **15**, 4, 390–405.

Carpenter M (1977) Managerialism and the division of labour in nursing. In *Readings in the Sociology of Nursing* (eds R Dingwall and J McIntosh). Edinburgh: Churchill Livingstone.

Choon G and Skevington S (1992) How do women and men in nursing perceive each other? In *Research and practice: A reader for nurses and the caring professions* (eds P Abbot and R Sapsford). Buckingham: Open University Press.

Darbyshire P (1986) The Unfairer Sex. *Senior Nurse*, **5**, 516, 44–46.

Dingwall R (1972) Nursing: Towards a Male Dominated Profession? *Nursing Times*, **68**, 41, 1294–95.

Dingwall R and McIntosh J (eds) (1978) *Readings in the Sociology of Nursing*. Edinburgh: Churchill Livingstone.

Dolan B (1990) Project 2000: The Gender Mender. *Nursing Standard*, **4**, 47, 52–3.

Garmarnikow E (1991) Nurse or Woman: Gender and Professionalism in Reformed Nursing 1860–1923. In *Nursing and Anthroplogy*, (eds P Holen and J Littlewood). London: Routledge.

Gaze H (1987) Men in nursing. *Nursing Times*, **83**, 20, 25–7.

Goody J (1982) *Cooking, Cuisine and Class*. Cambridge: Cambridge University Press.

Hardy K (1987) Career politics: the case of career histories of selected leading female and male nurses in England and Scotland. In *Political Issues in Nursing: Past Present and Future* Vol. 2 (ed R White). Chichester: John Wiley.

Hase S (1977) The role of the man in nursing. *Australian Nurses' Journal Review*, **7**, 1, 52.

Hass C (1977) Nursing — The Female Profession? *International Nursing Review*, **24**, 6, 166–7.

Henderson V (1966) *The Nature of Nursing*. London: Collier Macmillan.

Hutt R (1985) *Chief Nursing Officer Career Profiles: A Study of Backgrounds*. Brighton: Institute of Management Studies.

Jones M (1984) An investigation into attitudes towards men in nursing, with a particular emphasis on female patient care. Unpublished BSc (Hons) Nursing Dissertation. London: Polytechnic of South Bank.

Kalisch P A and Kalisch B J (1982) Nursing on prime time television. *American Journal of Nursing*, **82**, 2, 264–70.

Lancet Commission on Nursing (1932) Final Report. London: *Lancet*.

Littlewood R (1991) Gender, Role, Sickness: The Ritual Psychopathologies of the Nurse. In *Anthropology and Nursing* (eds P Holden and J Littlewood). London: Routledge.

Marrow C (1990) Points of View. *Nursing Standard*, **5**, 6, 41.

Marx K (1867) *Capital — A Critique of Political Economy*. Moscow: Progress Press.

McAllen D L (1961) Status of the Male Nurse. *Hospital Progress*, **41**, 61.

McKay L (1989) *Nursing a Problem*. Milton Keynes: Open University Press.

Ministry of Health, Scottish Home and Health Department (1966) *The Report of the Committee on Senior Nursing Staff Structure*. London: HMSO (Salmon Report).

Moccia P (1988) At the faultline: social activism and caring. *Nursing Outlook*, **36**, 1, 30–3.

Osborne R J (1989) Why do the Trade Unions do so little for Women? (Unpublished).

Pearson A (1992) Knowing nursing: emerging paradigms in nursing. In *Knowledge for Nursing Practice* (eds K Robinson and B Vaughan). Oxford: Butterworth–Heinemann.

Royal College of Nursing (1989) *Don't Divide Health Care* Campaign Pack. London: RCN.

Salvage J (1985) *Politics of Nursing*. London: Heinemann Nursing.

Sheehy G (1976) *Passages*. New York: E P Dutton.

TUC (1947) *Annual Report*. London: TUC.

Webb C. (1985) *Sexuality, Nursing & Health*. Chichester: Wiley.

Wright S (1991) Facilitating Therapeutic Nursing and Independent Practice. In *Nursing as Therapy* (eds A Pearson and S McMahon). London: Chapman and Hall.

CHAPTER 7

A Reflection on Issues for Practice

Pippa Gough, Sian Maslin-Prothero and Abigail Masterson

'Nursing is, quite simply, a practice, but its practice is far from simple.'
(Pearson, 1992)

INTRODUCTION

The aim of this chapter is to explore the potential impact of Project 2000 (UKCC 1986) on clinical practice. This may seem somewhat premature in that, at the time of writing, very few qualified 'knowledgeable doers', Project 2000 style, exist. It is nevertheless, possible to discuss the impact on clinical care from a broader perspective. This involves drawing together material from diverse sources, including experiences from nursing colleagues abroad, UK graduate programmes and the deluge of comment and speculation in the professional literature. The discussion will focus on a number of key themes and their implications for clinical practice, namely: the pursuit of intellectualism; inequalities and recruitment issues; affiliation to Higher Education (HE); teacher development; clinical experience; single level registration; and post-registration opportunities. Special consideration will be given to clinical practice in the community as it is envisaged that this is the area where the greatest impact on practice will occur — in light of the new practitioner being qualified, for the first time, to work in both institutional and non-institutional settings. The urgent need for concentrated research into the effects of both the change in preparation and the new practitioner on patient/client care will be exposed.

THE PURSUIT OF INTELLECTUALISM

One of the key motivations behind Project 2000 was a vision of the nurse as a knowledgeable doer and enabler, better equipped to respond to the health needs of the future (UKCC 1986). The new nurse education and preparation aims to encourage nurses to embrace and build upon a body of knowledge which can inform and improve practice (Orr 1987). This enhanced and more secure knowledge base has been seen as vital to an increase in nursing confidence, skills and autonomy (Robinson 1991b; Clark 1991; White 1988). To date, research in this area has supported this contention (Leonard and Jowett 1990). In their study of Project 2000 pilot sites, these authors found that the students appeared to learn more quickly, nurse with more sensitivity and communicate more effectively than those from more traditional courses. This reflects Benner's (1984) work, which shows nursing to be a highly complex activity, requiring sophisticated, high level preparation.

However, this pursuit of greater knowledge for nurses has not been globally endorsed. The major criticisms come pejoratively from within its own ranks and, unsurprisingly perhaps, the medical profession. Some nurses have argued that a need for intellectualism for a profession which is practice-based is artificial and elitist (Swaffield 1988; *Nursing Times* 1992a). Interestingly, Loos and Maddox (1989) discovered that even graduate nurses in Canada were not particularly enthusiastic about raising the academic level of the entire profession — which the authors attribute to being the result of a perceived loss of status amongst a present elite. To a certain extent elitism is inevitable, but as Robinson (1988) asserts, this is not necessarily deleterious to the profession.

It would appear that doctors are the group most challenged and threatened by greater academic credibility for nurses, both in the UK (*British Medical Journal* 1987; Hayward 1991; Devlin 1987; Gibberd 1988), and in other countries. When the initial report (UKCC 1986) was published, the power of the medical establishment was brought to bear on the government in an attempt to stop Project 2000 becoming reality (Orr 1988). Devlin (op. cit.) and the *BMJ* (op. cit.) both complain that the UKCC failed to consult doctors sufficiently about their views on a change in nurse education. They go on to rehearse the now familiar litany that the new education would be elitist and undesirable, not necessarily making better nurses, who are after all involved in a practical job which does not require academic foundation. The suggestion is the increased focus on academia may lead to a paucity of clinical skills. This fear however has not been realised with regard to the graduate experience (Sinclair 1983). Orr (1987) condemns this backward thinking of our health colleagues, which she describes as a double standard which implies:

'. . . while the education of nurses is best carried out as part of giving nursing care, the same criteria do not apply to the teaching of medicine.' (p. 24)

This professional infighting, as illustrated by the vociferous response (Brandon 1991; Brewin 1991; Hayward 1991; Norcross 1991) to Clark's (1991) letter to the *BMJ* seeking acknowledgement by the medical profession of the intellectual component of nursing, is not the most effective way to respond adequately to a growing and changing demand for health care. A more optimistic and constructive approach is offered by Christman (1988). Both he and Clark (op. cit.) contend that with the growing affiliation of nursing to the academic domain, the overlap of knowledge and competency with other disciplines — particularly the medical profession — will increase as pre-registration education for nurses intensifies. Ultimately this will create a growing homogeneity in the preparation of health professionals and will:

'. . . lessen the suspicion of others, soften communication barriers, offset tendencies towards territoriality and promote the growth of shared power.' (p. 4)

Christman (op. cit.) sees this parity with other professionals as central to nurses being able to access and influence decision making at a level that formulates policy and allocates resources. This is surely an important goal of Project 2000 education and one with the most significant impact on clinical practice. That is, the goal of enabling nurses to be proactive, rather than reactive, in the provision of care within the broader socio-economic environment.

PERPETUATING INSTITUTIONALISED INEQUALITIES?

The debate concerning the pursuit of intellectualism is not, however, the only contentious issue in respect of an enhanced knowledge base for nursing. Criticism has also been voiced with regard to the quality and content of the new Project 2000 curricula, namely that the knowledge being pursued is fundamentally flawed. In 1986, Safder Mohammed was one of the first to comment on the poor recognition given by Project 2000 to black people and minority ethnic groups in British society, a fact which has since attracted frequent and angry comment by a number of authors (Baxter 1988; Kings Fund 1989; Akinsanya 1988). Mohammed (op. cit.) argues the new preparation ignored the fact that 3.2 per cent of Britain's population at that time was black. By virtue of marginalising issues to do with race and equality of opportunity, Project 2000 is guilty of proposing an inappropriate and inadequate education. If the curriculum remains fundamentally racist, there can be no hope for a change in clinical practice in this direction.

Concerns have also been raised with regard to racist practices in recruitment to nursing. In July 1991 a letter from the registrar of UKCC (Ralph 1991) drew the profession's attention to:

'. . . the need to ensure that applicants from black and minority backgrounds are not disadvantaged in their quest for entry into programmes of education, leading to registration.' (p. 1)

The black communities in Britain have played a major role in the building and maintenance of the NHS. However they continue to be concentrated in unskilled, low status and poorly paid positions within this organisation (Doyal *et al.* 1980; Akinsanya 1988; Baxter 1988; Kings Fund 1990a and b). For nursing this means that black people are over-represented in nursing auxiliary and enrolled nurse posts (Equal Opportunities Commission 1991). This is compounded by racism in initial education resulting in fewer black people achieving the necessary educational entry requirements for nursing (Swann Committee 1985; Baxter op. cit.). Because Project 2000 proposes discontinuation of enrolled nurse programmes and the pursuit of only one level of qualified nurse — without resourcing structured programmes to make access for all groups a reality — there is a real danger that the position of nursing as a white middle-class profession will be perpetuated (COHSE 1986). This vicious cycle of discrimination is reflected in the experience of countries such as Australia that have already made this transition to higher education (Neill and Barclay 1989).

Baxter (op. cit.) notes that the numbers of black people entering nursing education courses are already falling and identifies racism as being the major cause. A considerable amount has been written about the projected shortfall in the number of 18 year olds (CBI 1988) although the NHS Regional Manpower (*sic*) Planners' Group have identified that black youth in this age range is in fact increasing. However, in order to target this group, specific attention must be paid to promoting genuine equal opportunity policies in the NHS which will enable fuller and fairer access.

The above situation begs the question, how can Project 2000 claim to produce nurses who will provide racially and culturally sensitive care, unless deep-seated attitudes are changed? The solution may lie in the wider use of ethnic monitoring, the destruction of racist stereotypes and positive action as stipulated in the Race Discrimination Act (1976). Recent reports from the King's Fund (1990a and b; 1988) and other writers such as Akinsanya (1988) argue this is the only way for black people to begin to challenge institutional racism and to educate health service workers about the actual needs and requirements of the British black and ethnic minority communities. Those few black nurses who have made it to the higher echelons are not 'honorary whites' or the product of tokenism. They do in fact continue to experience racial discrimination and have got to the top by virtue of hard work and are deserving of this status (Akinsanya 1990).

Equality of opportunity, however, is not only concerned with issues of race. Ralph (1991) also states the need to select a variety of nursing students:

'. . . drawn from a rich mix of age, background and talents to reflect the diversity of the population for which they will ultimately be caring.' (p. 1)

Within this category attention has been focused on the mature entrant, in particular within Project Paper 9 (UKCC 1987) which suggested recruitment of this group should be increased by 1000 per year following establishment of the new programme. Strategies to recruit from this section of the population, however, appear to have been neglected in the race to establish the new curriculum. Buchan, in a study done in 1991, found little difference in the composition of Project 2000 and traditional cohorts in this respect (he also found little change in the ratio of men to women entrants).

Assumptions seem to have been made about the appeal of the broader curriculum to mature entrants without taking into consideration practical arrangements to meet their needs, for example part-time and flexible learning opportunities and adequate child care facilities. The expectation is that mature students will adapt to the new diploma course and not vice versa. At least one college of nursing in the authors' experience has dismantled an innovative programme specifically tailored to the needs of mature entrants, in favour of whole-scale adoption of a Project 2000 common foundation programme. Nurse education, and thus clinical practice, will be the poorer as a result. Additionally it is still unclear whether issues of educational and personal support, particularly for those students for whom English is not a first language or who have been out of education for some time, are being adequately addressed.

Elsewhere in this book, Dolan and Allen have explored in more detail the implications for the profession of having more men and mature entrants into nursing.

LINKS WITH HIGHER EDUCATION (HE)

Many claims have been advanced regarding the benefits of the linking of nurse education with the actual institutions of higher education (HE). Wilson-Barnett (cited in Bailey 1990) contrasted the positive focus in HE on the abilities of the individual with the classic nursing focus on safety, uniformity and following of rules. Leonard and Jowett (1990) comment on the increase in the confidence of teaching staff that HE links facilitated, and Morle (1989) welcomes the opportunity to end educational isolation. Robinson (1991a) states many potential benefits have already been identified in one of the Project 2000 demonstration districts, in particular additional specialised resources and expertise, increased academic credibility and cross-fertilisation of ideas.

However, warnings have been sounded with regard to the take-over of nursing by HE. It is feared that control of the professional curriculum may be lost, and with it a nursing led preparation for practice. Chapman (1990), for example, notes that colleges of nursing in their eagerness to be accepted by HE have been prepared to agree to almost any proposal for affiliation or amalgamation. This need to retain autonomy within HE has been highlighted in Australia by Gruending (1989), who describes the way nursing can be subsumed by the larger, potentially more powerful disciplines — a consequence of which is non-nurses making decisions about nursing curricula and programmes.

Collins (1990) stresses the need for an integrated approach in all aspects of planning and provision, citing as an example that a particular sociological perspective is necessary for the nursing student (such as that outlined by Perry 1991), rather than simply being included in part of an undergraduate course in sociology.

Addditionally, there is the problem of the physical isolation of most colleges of nursing from the HE institutions. One of the main aims of Project 2000, as Chapman (op. cit.) points out, was to involve nursing students more fully in student and campus life generally. Simpson *et al.* (1979) showed undergraduate nursing students, despite having full nursing status and access to all student activities, tended to remain isolated. If the present practice of keeping nursing students in a separate building, often miles from the main campus and all its resources, persists, how will the benefits of integration be realised?

If nurse students and teachers are apart from the mainstream of HE, their influence on the future direction of such education is likely to be limited. Nursing must ensure it is an equal partner in policy making at all levels, if, ultimately, clinical practice is to reflect a knowledge base appropriate to nursing.

TEACHER DEVELOPMENT

As Charlwood has already shown in Chapter 4, and has been noted above, a move into HE can provide a considerable boost to nurse teacher confidence, it can also provoke a fair amount of stress due to the mammoth changes in approach and philosophy required. Not only must nurse teacher preparation courses recognise these tensions, but the situation suggests the need for ongoing teacher development programmes to be established with some urgency. This point is elaborated by Tuddenham and Beacock (1989), who suggest that in order to gain the advantages of an HE model the relevant educational culture needs to be nurtured.

Mason (1991) questions, for example, whether it is in fact an easy matter for the principles of self-directed learning to be assimilated by teaching staff who are products of more rigid systems. Darbyshire (1991) succinctly pursues this point in his suggestion that for the Project 2000 'revolution' to become reality nurse educators must have imagination and creativity — a situation he finds impossible to envisage within current approaches to nurse teacher preparation. An HMI report (1989) showed that teachers were having problems successfully managing large group teaching (70–100 students) and indicated the need to review teaching methods, again emphasising the necessity of adequate staff development.

(This is often compounded by the lack of adequate room available in many colleges of nursing.)

Another major implication for nurse teachers is the move into the health based curriculum, which has often been foreign territory for teachers educated themselves within a disease model. In fact, students themselves are increasingly commenting on the discomfort with which this health emphasis is managed within colleges across the country (Allen 1992).

Teacher development was also identified as a key issue in changing to an HE model in Israel (Bevis and Krulik 1991) — a situation which was remedied by the intensification of continuing education for nurse teachers to enable this transition. The UKCC (1987) did point out the need for appropriate education and reorientation for teachers and stated that provision for this must be built into Project 2000 implementation plans. However, there appears to be little evidence of this to date. Unfortunately this situation does not augur well for the envisaged advancement of nursing practice, as outlined in the initial Project 2000 proposals. If the positive suggestions put forward by the English National Board (ENB 1989) for 'managing change' in nurse education, are pursued more vigorously, a successful shift may well be achieved, thus facilitating excellence in clinical practice.

CLINICAL EXPERIENCE

Nursing, as frequently stated, is a practice-based profession and quality of practice ultimately hinges on appropriate and rewarding clinical placements. Many of these ideas have been developed from the seminal works of Ogier (1982) and Fretwell (1982) who identified that learning pejoratively takes place in practice areas. However, concern has increasingly been expressed regarding the availability and quality of clinical experience, especially in the light of Project 2000 and current changes wrought by the NHS reforms (Fardell 1989; Tuddenham and Beacock 1989; Carlisle 1990). These concerns are also reflected by authors examining similar practice changes in their own countries, in particular Sherrard (1990) in New Zealand and Ives and Rowley (1990) in Australia. Fardell (1989) focuses on NHS Trusts which she suggests may find the provision of clinical placements too time consuming and expensive, whilst Tuddenham and Beacock (1989) highlight the extreme pressure on placement areas from Business Technician and Education Council (BTech) and Health Care Assistant courses and Youth

Training Schemes. Carlisle (1991) has also suggested that colleges may soon have to pay for placements. The importance of access to relevant clinical areas cannot be overemphasised if diplomates are to gain the necessary skills for improved professional practice, the ultimate aim of Project 2000.

There is also a concern that these placements may be weakened even further by the demise of the clinical teacher. The major load of clinical teaching and supervision now falls on the shoulders of clinical staff. But are these staff the most appropriate to teach future practitioners? Brown (1988) notes that where nursing has failed in the past is in the assumption that proficiency in nursing equates with proficiency in teaching nursing skills. Although tacit learning is important, a 'sitting by Nellie' approach is not enough. If nursing is to achieve the 'new dawn' as promised in Project 2000 (UKCC 1986), the use of existing role models alone is insufficient. Leonard and Jowett (1990), in their study of Project 2000 pilot sites, emphasise the need for conscious development of the teaching role of qualified staff and go on to advocate supernumeracy for mentors — an unlikely development in today's financial climate. It could also be argued that a supernumerary mentor is, in fact, a clinical teacher by any other name.

In some areas the role of lecturer–practitioner is being strongly advocated as a means of resolving the problem of appropriate clinical supervision (Vaughan 1989; Clifford 1989) and where the development of the role is clearly understood, it has been highly successful (Vaughan 1989). However, supporters of this approach warn it is not only a structural, but also an attitudinal change that is required and therefore cannot be indiscriminately adopted (ibid).

Leonard and Jowett (1990), echoing Melia's (1987) earlier work, also identify, somewhat worryingly, that the pressure to conform to existing nursing values overrides any positive effect of supervision and clinical teaching. They found students:

'. . . rapidly discovering that practice assessment depended on their relationship with the ward staff [and so] made it their business to get on with the ward staff.' (p. 19)

Even if this was at the expense of developing the qualities the diploma scheme set out to nurture. As Turner and Dickson (1988) indicate, a change of attitude is required among existing nurses in order to prevent the diploma student from feeling alienated and thus wanting to conform. Thomas (1989), in relation to graduate nurses, argued that if traditional nurses could only accept and expect these students to be different and to possess different skills, then change could occur — a point that is perhaps equally relevant to the Project 2000 students and associated promises of improved practice.

Hopes have been pinned on the move to HE creating an assertive nurse, and breaking the mould of submissiveness that has dogged nursing for so long. In Canada, however, despite a whole-scale shift into HE, a study showed nursing students were significantly more submissive and less willing to lead and innovate than other HE students (Dych *et al.* 1991). This trend to conformity might well inhibit the use of Project 2000 learners as catalysts for change and is unlikely to be overcome by affiliation to HE institutions alone. However, if the cultural shift among nurse teachers can be achieved, as discussed above, then a more positive role model is available to help break this mould of submissiveness. At the end of the day, clinical practice must benefit.

SINGLE REGISTRATION NURSING

Implicit in Project 2000 is the idea of the single level of registered practitioner. Mason (1991) and Clifford (1989) fear that an unintended consequence of Project 2000, far from ultimately resulting in one level of nurse, may well create unhelpful divisions between differently prepared nurses, making any positive changes unlikely. This is particularly so in the light of the rapidly growing population of Health Care Assistants and the potential fragmentation of the profession implied by PREPP (UKCC 1990) and ENB Framework (1990). There have been worrying reports of students on existing courses feeling resentful and bitter with regard to their Project 2000 colleagues (*Nursing Standard* 1990) — an issue reflected in the earlier discussion on acceptance of diploma students in the clinical areas. Despite the UKCC's assurances to the contrary, the fear is that non-diploma registered nurses (RN) will not be able to compete effectively in an open market against the diplomates. In these circumstances how ethical is it still to be offering RN training within an already demoralised workforce. By any account, the effect on clinical practice cannot be positive. These issues need to be urgently addressed if they are not to blight what is otherwise a positive force for change.

The plight of the Enrolled Nurse also deserves consideration here. Twenty years after Briggs (HMSO 1972) and the recommendation

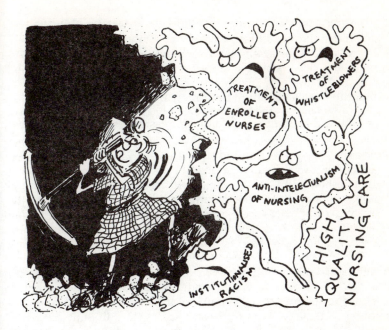

that enrolled nurse training should cease — a proposal which was central to Project 2000 — Buchan (1991) reports that 591 students entered this training in England in 1990. This situation is surely highly unethical, especially considering that not only is their access to Project 2000 courses on the whole prohibited and entrance to conversion courses limited (many of which are not even at diploma level), but also their future employment prospects look extremely bleak (*Nursing Times* 1992b). This is in spite of the UKCC (1987) recommendation that opportunities for continuing education for this group be exploited and developed and that funds for this should be specifically identified. Recent initiatives, particularly in the field of open and distance learning such as the Royal College of Nursing *Nursing Standard*'s Nursing Update, the *Nursing Times* Open Learning programme and other similar ventures, are positive attempts to improve the situation.

POST-REGISTRATION OPPORTUNITIES

Whilst enrolled nurses have been marginalised in terms of their professional development, it has nevertheless been argued that the key to the success of Project 2000 is the preparation and enhancement of existing practitioners as well as the need for realistic continuing education programmes (Spencer 1989; Ryall Davies and Wainwright 1989; Lathlean *et al.* 1986; Brown 1988; Bolger 1990). Despite this, the continued dearth of post-registration opportunities has been widely documented both here, and also abroad (Loos and Maddox 1989; Morle 1989; Orr 1990b). To a certain extent the Post-registration Education and Practice Project (PREPP) (UKCC 1990), and the English National Board (ENB) Framework for Continuing Professional Education (ENB 1990) can be seen as an attempt to resolve this situation. The implications of further dissecting the profession through the introduction of advanced practitioner and consultant nurse levels, however, in the view of these authors remains a subject of conjecture. Whatever the outcome, serious concerns are already being voiced regarding the commitment of existing employers to necessary time and funding required and the overall philosophy of academic development of nurses. Additionally, the biggest single failing of both PREPP and the ENB Framework has been that these recommendations should have been implemented before the commencement of Project 2000, if real change was to have been achieved. Nevertheless, it is comforting to note that Leonard and Jowett (1990) did find that nursing staff were 'kept on their toes' by the diploma students, and were motivated to make more use of learning resources and libraries. It would seem, therefore, that even without structured post-registration education programmes, staff are spontaneously seeking to improve their knowledge base in line with Project 2000, thus enhancing clinical practice.

THE COMMUNITY CONTEXT

Finally, the impact of Project 2000 on clinical practice within the community context is perhaps the most considerable. To date, not only has the new preparation sparked intense debate on the education and future form of community nursing, culminating in the Community Education and Practice (CEP) proposals (UKCC 1991), but it has also begun to have a number of implications for the current workloads and practice of post-qualified nurses in non-institutional settings.

Initially, following the publication of project paper 9 (UKCC 1987), community nurses expressed alarm that the new practitioner would be able to practise not only within institutions but also in 'non-institutional' settings without further preparation (Batchelor and Cofield 1989; Whitney 1989; Orr 1991). Prior to this, community nurses in all disciplines had been increasingly required to undertake further training and education in order to assume responsibility for care in community clinical areas. Yet this paper suggested that the diploma-prepared nurse would be competent to do the same from initial registration.

Batchelor and Cofield (1989) compared the Project 2000 curriculum with district nurse preparation and concluded that, on paper, the new breed of nurse could function fairly well in both settings, if curricula were the only consideration. However, they argued this was not the only point at issue. There were also concerns that, within the context of the wider community, the new Project 2000 preparation would not necessarily have equipped the diplomate with the maturity and professional confidence required to initiate structured programmes of care and appropriately delegate work to support staff.

In 1991, the UKCC Community Education and Practice (CEP) working party reflected this thinking, by suggesting that the Project 2000 nurse would be a valuable addition to the community team but only under the leadership of an appropriately prepared 'community health care nurse'. The report quite clearly acknowledges that the complexity of work within the community arena will continue to require nurses with specialist skills and knowledge (ibid). Within these terms of reference, the impact of Project 2000 on community clinical practice can be seen to be the development of an increasing diversity of community nursing, able to respond more effectively to the health needs of the future.

Although it has now been recognised that the new practitioner will not immediately be a 'specialist' within the non-institutional setting, she or he will nevertheless be better equipped to work in this environment than are her more traditionally educated colleagues. After all, Project 2000 does offer a greatly enhanced education based on a health model and closely focused on health promotion. Correspondingly, as Orr (1990a) points out, the Project 2000 student will need a different form of community experience — and this has major implications for the workloads and clinical practice of existing staff in the field. Ayton (1988) explored this fact in relation to health visitors and highlighted the need for more in-service training on teaching and assessing skills, the forming of closer links with educationalists and the increase in time devoted to the organisation of relevant community programmes and student assessment, all of which were seen to have drastic service implications. Ayton (ibid) suggested the need for a 2.5 per cent increase in establishment to cope with this increase in workload. However, in today's reality of financial constraint and tenuous employment futures, this seems an unlikely eventuality for existing health visitors. Consequently clinical practice is bound to be affected, but it is difficult to say whether this under-resourcing really outweighs the positive benefits of this long awaited new education.

CONCLUSION

This chapter has explored a number of key issues in relation to Project 2000 in an attempt to determine their effect on clinical practice. Much of the impetus behind the push for Project 2000 has been the consistent finding both in the UK and the USA that the better educated nurses are, the better the standard of clinical practice (Krauss 1990; Wilson-Barnett cited in Bailey 1990). It appears, however, that the issues are somewhat more complex than this statement would lead us to believe. The pursuit of intellectualism, although arguably covetable, is not wholeheartedly supported either intra- or inter-professionally. Recruitment is far from ideal in terms of equality of access and equality of opportunity. Links with HE have already raised a number of problems, not least of which is the apparent lessening of decision-making power. Opportunities for development of both teachers and existing practitioners in all areas and at all levels, must be pursued as a matter of great urgency, in order to avoid further demoralisation and fragmentation of the workforce. Ultimately, Project 2000 will succeed if it can show that the benefit to the patient is paramount. The only way this can be ascertained is through extensive research, carried out by nurses and for nurses and firmly grounded in practice.

REFERENCES

Akinsanya J A (1990) Tokenism in nursing, *Nursing Standard*, 5, 13/14, 48.
Akinsanya J A (1988) Ethnic minority nurses, midwives and health visitors: What role for them in the NHS? *New Community*, **XIV**, 5.
Allen C (1992) Foundation for success. *Nursing Times*, **88**, 2, 20.
Ayton M (1988) Health Visitors Supplement 'Defining a key role'. *Nursing Times*, **84**, 42, 76–7.
Bailey L (1990) Practising to win. *Nursing Standard*, 5, 1, 20.
Batchelor S and Cofield M (1989) Beyond Project 2000. *Journal of District Nursing* 8, 4, 19–20.
Baxter C (1988) *The Black Nurse: An Endangered Species, a Case for Equal Opportunities in Nursing*. Cambridge: National Extension College.
Benner P (1984) *From novice to expert: excellence and power in clinical practice*. Menlo Park: Addison Wesley.

Bevis E O and Krulik I T (1991) Nationwide Faculty Development: a model for a shift from Diploma to Baccalaureate education. *Journal of Advanced Nursing*, 16, 3, 362–70.

BMJ (1987) Final Proposals on Project 2000. *British Medical Journal*, **294**, 458.

Bolger T (1990) Could do better. *Nursing Times*, **86**, 13, 31–2.

Brandon S (1991) Letters. *British Medical Journal*, **303**, 580.

Brewin T (1991) Letters, *British Medical Journal*, **303**, 580.

Brown M (1988) Better get ready! *Nursing Times*, **84**, 35, 53–4.

Buchan J (1991) Characteristics of student cohorts. *Nursing Standard*, **5**, 52, 25.

Carlisle D (1990) Pay as you learn. *Nursing Times*, **87**, 44, 22.

Chapman C (1990) Selling nursing short. *Nursing Standard*, **4**, 29, 51.

Christman L P (1988) A conceptual model for centers of excellence in nursing. *Nurse Administration Quarterly*, **12**, 4, 1–4.

Clark J (1991) On these rocks . . . commitment to nurse education in 1990's. *Nursing Practice*, **4**, 2, 2–6.

Clark J (1991) Nursing: an intellectual activity. *British Medical Journal*, **303**, 376–7.

Clifford C (1989) Project 2000: Clinical practice and continuing education. *Nursing Standard*, **3**, 46, 42–5.

Collins S (1990) Occasional Paper: The ENB pilot schemes: how plans have become reality. *Nursing Times*, **86**, 31, 30–3.

Confederation of British Industry (1988) *Workforce 2000: An agenda for action*. London: CBI.

Confederation of Health Service Employees (1986) *COHSE's Response to the UKCC Document "Project 2000: a new preparation for practice"*. Banstead: COHSE.

Darbyshire P (1991) The American Revolution. *Nursing Times,* **87**, 6, 57–8.

Devlin B (1987) 'An unreal brave new world? *Nursing Times*, **83**, 18, 29–30.

Doyal L, Hunt G and Mellor J (1980) Your life in their hands: migrant workers in the national health service. *Critical Social Policy* Autumn, **2**, 54–71.

Dych S *et al.* (1991) Entry and Exit Characteristics of Baccalaureate Nursing Students. *The Canadian Journal of Nursing Research*, **23**, 1, 27–40.

ENB (1989) *Managing Change in Nursing Education*, London: ENB.

ENB (1990) *Framework for Continuing Professional Education and Training for Nurses, Midwives and Health Visitors*. London: ENB.

Equal Opportunities Commission (1991) *Equality Management: Women's Employment in the NHS*. Manchester: EOC.

Fardell J (1989) Project 2000: envisaging education. *Nursing Times*, **85**, 37, 31–2.

Fretwell J E (1992) *Ward Teaching and Learning*. London: RCN.

Gibberd B (1988) Project 2000 – The Only Option? *The Health Service Journal*, **98**, 182–3.

Gruending D L (1989) Nursing Education in Australia. Canadienne Nurse/ Infirmière **85**, 11, 30–31.

Hayward S A (1991) Letter to the editor. *British Medical Journal*, **303**, 580.

HMI (1989) *A Survey of Collaboration in Nurse Education in Four Polytechnics and Colleges*, Autumn, Middlesex: Department of Education and Science.

HMSO (1972) *Report on the Committee on Nursing*. London: HMSO, (Briggs Report).

Ives G and Rowley G (1990) A clinical learning milieu: nurse clinicians' attitudes to tertiary education and teaching. *The Australian Journal of Advanced Nursing*, **7**, 4, 29–35.

King Edward's Hospital Fund for London (1990a) *Racial Equality: the Nursing Profession* (Equal Opportunity Task Force Occasional Paper Number 6). London: King's Fund.

King Edward's Hospital Fund for London (1990b) *Ethnic Minority Health Authority Membership: a Survey*. London: King's Fund.

King Edward's Hospital Fund for London (1989) *Equal Opportunities Employment Policies in the NHS: Ethnic Monitoring*. London: King's Fund.

Krauss J (1990) Education and experience . . . part 2. *Nursing Standard*, **4**, 15, 20–1.

Lathlean J *et al.* (1986) *Professional Development Schemes for Newly Registered Nurses* Summary of Findings, Conclusions and Recommendations of the Evaluation Project. London: University of London.

Leonard A and Jowett S (1990) *Charting the Course: A study of the six Pilot Schemes in Pre-registration Nurse Education Research Paper Number 1*. London: National Foundation for Educational Research.

Loos C and Maddox K (1989) Baccalaureate Nurses: Territoriality and Professionalism. *The Canadian Journal of Nursing Research*, **21**, 3, 19–29.

Mason C (1991) Project 2000: a critical review. *Nursing Practice*, **4**, 3, 2–5.

Melia K (1987) *Learning and Working: the Occupational Socialism of Nurses*. London: Tavistock.

Mohammed S (1986) A black perspective. *Senior Nurse*, **5**, 3, 5.

Morle K (1989) Where nursing education should be based. *Nursing Standard*, **3**, 25, 25–8.

Neill J and Barclay L (1989) Sociodemographic characteristics of nursing students in higher education. *The Australian Journal of Advanced Nursing*, **7**, 1, 4–11.

Norcross K (1991) Letters. *British Medical Journal*, **303**, 580.

Nursing Standard (1990) Student anger focuses on Project 2000 changeover, **4**, 24, 5.

Nursing Times (1992a) Letters: how to lose the new nurses. *Nursing Times*, **88**, 9, 15.

Nursing Times (1992b) Letters: conversion let-down. *Nursing Times*, **88**, 1, 10–11.

Ogier M E (1982) *An Ideal Sister: A study of learning styles and verbal interactions of ward sisters and nurse learners in general hospital*. London: RCN.

Orr J (1987) Why shouldn't we be clever? *Nursing Times*, **83**, 35, 24.

Orr J (1988) Enemies of Project 2000. *Nursing Times*, **84**, 44, 24.

Orr J (1990a) Tradition v Project 2000 — something old, something new. *Nurse Education Today*, **10**, 1, 58–62.

Orr J (1990b) Project 2000 and the specialist practitioner. *Nursing Standard*, **4**, 17, 35–7.

Orr J (1991) Facing the challenge. *Nursing*, **4**, 44, 25–7.

Perry A (1991) Sociology — its contributions and critiques. In: *Nursing: A Knowledge Base for Practice*. Perry A and Jolley M (eds) London: Edward Arnold.

Ralph C (1991) *Registrar's Letter: Equality of Opportunity. Entry into Programmes of Nursing, Midwifery and Health Visiting Education*. London: UKCC.

Robinson J (1988) Elitism in Nursing. *Nursing Times*, **84**, 40, 50–1.

Robinson J (1991a) Power, politics and policy analysis in nursing. In: *Nursing: A Knowledge Base for Practice* Perry A and Jolly M (eds) pp. 271–307, London: Edward Arnold.

Robinson J (1991b) Evaluating the courses. *Nursing Times*, **87**, 21, 29–30.

Ryall Davis and Wainwright P (1989) The shaping of Project 2000 in Wales. *Nursing Standard*, **3**, 32, 29–31.

Sherrard I (1990) Clinical Experience Vanishing. *New Zealand Nursing Journal* November, **83**, 5.

Simpson I H *et al.* (1979) *From student to nurse. A longitudinal study of socialisation*. Cambridge: Cambridge University Press.

Sinclair H C (1983) Graduate Nurses in the United Kingdom: Myth and Reality. *Nurse Education Today*, **7**, 1, 24–9.

Spencer D (1989) Project 2000: Demonstration. *Nursing Standard*, **4**, 13, 50–2.

Swaffield L (1988) Project 2000: the New Face of Nursing. *Nursing Times*, **84**, 31, 27–9.

Swann Committee (1985) *Education for all: The Report of the Committee of Inquiry into the Education of Children from Ethnic Minority Groups*. London: HMSO.

Thomas E (1989) Graduates' careers in nursing. *Nursing Standard*, **4**, 2, 45.

Tuddenham P and Beacock C (1989) The mental handicap branch for Project 2000. *Nursing Standard*, **3**, 40–3.

Turner T and Dickson N (1988) Project 2000: A New Dawn for Nursing? *Nursing Times*, **8**, 22, 12–13.

UKCC (1986) *Project 2000: A new preparation for practice*. London: UKCC.

UKCC (1987) *Project 2000 — The Final Proposals*. Project Paper 9. London: UKCC.

UKCC (1990) *The Report of the Post-Registration Education and Practice Project*. London: UKCC.

UKCC (1991) *Report on Proposals for the Future of Community Education and Practice*. London: UKCC.

Vaughan B (1989) Two Roles — one job. *Nursing Times*, **85**, 11, 52.

White R (1988) The influence of nursing on the politics of health. In *Political Issues in Nursing. Past, Present and Future, Vol. 3*. White R (ed). Chichester: John Wiley.

Whitney H (1989) Project 2000: The Implications for District Nursing and Health Visiting. *Nursing Standard*, **4**, 4, 30–3.

CHAPTER 8

Into the Community

June Clark

'Care in the community is a humane and supportive concept.'
(*Nursing Times* 1993)

More than a century before Project 2000, Florence Nightingale argued that 'hospitals are an intermediate stage of civilisation', and she 'looked to the day when there are no nurses to the sick but only nurses to the well' (Baly 1991). The reality is and always has been, that even when people are ill, only a tiny minority go to hospital, and when they do, they stay for a relatively short time. Most health care is provided in community settings where people live and work.

Traditionally however, this has not been reflected either in the way health care has been organised or in the way resources (money and people) have been deployed. In particular, most nurses have been employed in hospitals and their training (there has until now been relatively little *education*) has generally been operated in hospitals, by hospitals, and for hospitals.

Figure 8.1 shows the community's need for health care as a broad-based pyramid in which the greatest is at the broad base. Yet the pyramid which represents the deployment of nursing services is the exact opposite — its broad base is in hospitals. The nurse's educational experience is even more inappropriate — an even broader base in the hospital setting and only at the narrowest point does it dip into the area of greatest need.

A more appropriate framework for nursing is shown in Figure 8.2. The circle shows the five interrelated elements of the nurse's role in a comprehensive health service. The broad base of the pyramid

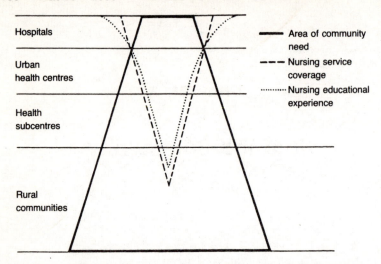

Figure 8.1 Existing nursing services related to community need and educational experience from: *Community Health Nursing*, Report of a WHO Expert Committee (WHO 1974).

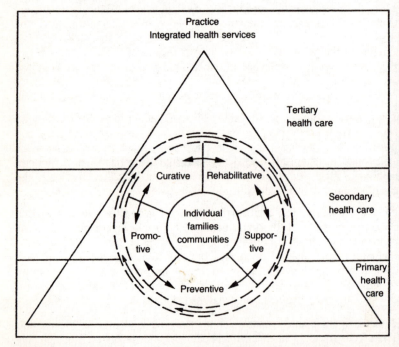

Figure 8.2 A conceptual framework for nursing from: *Review and Reorienting the Basic Nursing Curriculum* (WHO 1991).

is as in Figure 8.1 where most people need and receive their health care — thought not at present their nursing and medical care. All elements of the nurse's role are needed at all three levels of the pyramid; the arrows on the outside of the circle, however, indicate that no one element will assume permanent dominance. Each one will come to the fore at the appropriate time in response to the patient/client's particular needs, no matter what the setting.

Project 2000 challenges traditional attitudes and approaches to health care in many ways. This chapter is concerned with the realisation that if nurses are to make their full contribution to meeting people's health needs, their basic education must enable them to practise competently, not just in hospitals but in a range of institutional and non-institutional settings — wherever people *are*. As WHO has recently stated:

> 'The mission of nursing in society is to help individuals, families and groups to determine and achieve their physical, mental and social potential, and to do so within the challenging environment in which they live and work.' (WHO 1991a)

But the change which is required is not just about geographical settings, it involves a much more fundamental reorientation of practice, including new values, new skills and new ways of working — a shift towards primary health care.

PRIMARY HEALTH CARE — A RANGE OF SERVICES

Primary health care is not just the health services that are provided outside hospitals, nor just the kind of work done by general practitioners (who provide primary medical care) and specialist community nurses such as health visitors and district nurses, although this is the narrow definition which is often used in the UK. Nor is it a type of health care which is useful only for underserved populations in developing countries; it is as relevant in urban Britain as in Africa or Central America. It includes a range of services which are the first level of contact with a country's health care system; in the UK that means occupational health services, school nursing, retail pharmacists, child health clinics, as well as the work of the multi-disciplinary team based on general practice, and even some of the work (such as day care for elderly people and open-access outpatient clinics) which takes place in hospitals. It is not limited to the NHS, for such other sectors as environmental health, education, housing and nutrition are also important. WHO has defined eight elements as its essential components:

— education concerning prevailing health problems and methods of preventing and controlling them;
— the promotion of good food supply and proper nutrition;
— the provision of safe water and basic sanitation;
— maternal and child health care, including family planning;
— immunisation against the major infectious diseases;
— the prevention and control of locally endemic diseases;
— appropriate treatment of common diseases and injuries; and
— the provision of essential drugs.

All these services involve nurses, working as practitioners, teachers, organisers and policy makers — a far cry from the stereotypical images of frilly caps and the wards of acute general hospitals.

PRIMARY HEALTH CARE — A DIFFERENT PHILOSOPHY

Even more important, however, primary health care incorporates a particular philosophy and approach to health care which is based on five key principles:

— a focus on health and health promotion — promoting and maintaining health and preventing illness;
— community participation — involving individuals, families and communities in care and making it possible for them to take more responsibility for their health;
— equity — working actively to reduce inequities in access to health services and to meet the needs of groups and populations as well as individuals;
— multi-sectoral and multi-disciplinary collaboration — recognising the contribution to health of other sectors such as housing, education and nutrition working with others as partner in a multi-disciplinary team;
— appropriate technology — using methods, procedures, techniques and equipment which are scientifically valid, adapted to local needs and acceptable to those for whom they are used.

The differences between this approach and the more traditional approach to nursing practice are summarised in Table 8.1.

	Traditional nursing	Primary health care nursing
The patient	Sick or disabled individual seeking health care	Individuals, families and communities, sick or well
Nursing concepts	Diseases requiring curative treatment, especially in hospital	Prevailing health problems and needs of the community. Prevention of disease/disability, rehabilitations, care, support
Nursing interventions	'Basic' nursing care focused on people's physical needs: high-tech medically prescribed interventions aimed at cure	Teaching, counselling, mobilising coping mechanisms and self-care resources. Low-tech therapies aimed at rehabilitation and support as well as cure
Nursing role	Medical assistant	Member of multidisciplinary team
Preventive care	Focus on secondary prevention (e.g. screening) and tertiary prevention (e.g. rehabilitation)	Focus on primary prevention (health promotion, health teaching)
Place of practice	Hospitals and other institutions	Wherever people are
Learning environment for students	Hospitals and other institutions	Wherever people are

Source: adapted from WHO (1985) A guide to curriculum review for basic nursing education: orientation to primary health care and community health

Table 8.1   Comparison between traditional and primary health care orientations to nursing

HEALTH FOR ALL BY THE YEAR 2000

This reorientation of nursing practice is part of a major change in the direction of health policy which has been taking place in all countries of the world since the mid-1970's as part of the World Health Organisation's strategy for achieving Health for All by the Year 2000.

In 1977, the World Health Assembly resolved that

'the main social target of governments, international organisations and the whole world community in the coming decades should be the attainment by all peoples of the world by the year 2000 of a level of health that will permit them to lead a socially and economically productive life.' (WHO 1978)

The following year at a town called Alma Ata in the south eastern corner of what was then the USSR, all the member states of WHO signed a Declaration which identified primary health care as the key to achieving Health for All and called upon all governments to formulate national policies, strategies and plans of action to develop primary health care as the central focus of their health care system (WHO 1978). In 1983, the UK, along with the other countries of the European Region, agreed a strategy and an action plan, including 38 Targets for Health that describe the minimum progress that they must make by the year 2000 (WHO 1985).

Even before the Declaration of Alma Ata, nursing had already taken a lead by convening, in 1974, an Expert Committee on Community Health Nursing which had recognised that

'the provision of primary health care for all segments of the population is perhaps the most crucial health problem of most communities in the world today,'

and had made specific recommendations for reformulating nursing education to prepare all nurses for community nursing (WHO 1974). At the Alma Ata conference, the International Council of Nurses on behalf of its 97 member nursing associations, affirmed the commitment of nurses everywhere to the concepts and strategies of primary health care and their willingness to make the changes in nursing practice, education and management which are necessary for its achievement. In Europe, the Nursing Unit of the WHO Regional Office for Europe was already preparing for a European study on people's needs for nursing care; the study's main finding was the need to reorientate nursing practice in the light of the 38 Targets (WHO 1987). Accordingly, WHO convened the first European Conference on Nursing which was held in Vienna in 1989 (see Appendix III). The conference recommended that innovative nursing services should be developed which focus on health rather than disease; that, in keeping with European policies for Health for All, nursing practice should be based on the principles inherent in the primary health care approach; and that all basic programmes of nursing education should be restructured in order to produce nurses able to function in both hospital and community. Project 2000's recommendation that the new registered practitioner must be competent to practise in community as well as hospital settings is thus part of a world-wide movement in nursing.

'POWERHOUSE FOR CHANGE?'

The language of treaties and official documents is rarely inspirational but the excitement and challenge for nursing of the primary health care movement was captured in a now famous speech by Dr Halfdan Mahler, WHO's Director General:

> 'Millions of nurses throughout the world hold the key to an acceptance and expansion of primary health care because they work closely with people, whether they are community health nurses in the Amazon rain forests or intensive care nurses in a heart transplant unit. If the millions of nurses in a thousand different places articulate the same ideas and convictions about primary health care and come together as one force, they could act as a powerhouse for change. I believe that such a change is coming, and that nurses around the globe, whose work touches each of us intimately will greatly help to bring it about . . .

> The harnessing of nursing experience, energy, capabilities and commitment would add greatly to the momentum of primary health care development and would accelerate the achievement of the goal of Health for All.' (Mahler 1987)

The question is, how will nurses respond? Will Project 2000 give nurses the knowledge, attitudes and skills they will need to meet the challenge? Will the rhetoric become reality?

NURSING *IS* PRIMARY HEALTH CARE

One answer to these questions lies in the belief that

> 'to use the nurse as a major provider of primary health care requires no major extension of a function that is implicit in the definition of nursing.' (WHO 1982)

The definition of what is nursing is fundamental. A definition which is based on the prescriptive care of ill people in institutions is not compatible with the concepts of primary health care. However, when health rather than illness is recognised as a legitimate focus for nursing, and when nursing interventions shift from administering medically prescribed curative therapies towards teaching and enabling people to achieve for themselves their optimal level of health, the picture changes.

Such a shift is not new; it is 'radical' in the sense of 'a return to our roots'. As Miss Nightingale said:

> 'Every day, sanitary knowledge, or the knowledge of nursing or in other words, of how to put the constitution in such a state as that it will have no disease, or that it can recover from disease, takes a higher place. . . . The same laws of health or of nursing, for they are in reality the same, obtain among the well as among the sick.' (Baly 1991)

KNOWLEDGE AND SKILLS FOR COMMUNITY PRACTICE

Much of the skills and knowledge which are required for community practice are part of the stock in trade of the health visitor, school nurse and district nurse who have constituted the core of Britain's community health services for more than a century. More recently, they have been joined by new specialists in community nursing — community psychiatric nurses, nurses caring for people with learning disabilities, paediatric nurses, nurses working with particular client groups such as homeless people, and practice nurses. These nurses are the 'specialist practitioners' who Project 2000 envisages will be able to give professional advice and support to the first-level registered practitioner working in community settings. The UKCC report on proposals for the future of community education and practice (UKCC 1991) which sets out proposals for their education and training at post-registration level, makes clear that the Project 2000 registered practitioner will not be competent to practise as a community health nurse at this level without further training. What is needed is to identify the knowledge and skills which are necessary for primary practice in community settings and to ensure that these are part of pre-registration preparation.

Much of the knowledge base comes within the common foundation programme. Altschul (1989) argues:

> 'the common core of the syllabus for every one of the registers will be found in the community, not in hospital nursing. Health promotion, health education, prevention of illness must come first. Sociology, psychology, human biology, genetics and ethics are basic to all the caring professions. Nurses in all branches need to know about children, about families, about work and unemployment, about death and

bereavement; all nurses should be aware of the importance for health of economic well-being and the significance of stress whatever is causes. They need to discuss and think about the value systems of the society in which they live, about cultural differences, about the manifestations of ill-health when people find it difficult to adapt to events of importance in their life. There is enough material for the Common Foundation Programme without a student ever entering a hospital, though of course students should learn about the nature and place of these institutions in the health care system.' (Altschul 1989)

Her view that 'all hospital nursing courses should, I think, be post-registration courses' will seem extreme to traditionalists, but it is entirely in line with the Project 2000 view that

'there will always be a need for the hospital nurse, but as hospital nursing may well be much more the preserve of the specialist nurse in the year 2000, initial forms of preparation should take this into account.' (Project 2000 para 2.36); (UKCC 1986)

Many of the skills which have been traditionally the preserve of community nurses are important for all nurses and they need to be learned early. These skills include:

— communicating with all kinds of people in all kinds of settings;
— working in partnership with patients and informal carers;
— assessing environments not merely the individuals within them;
— working in unstructured environments and making decisions without immediate reference to colleagues or peers;
— ensuring continuity of care in the nurse's absence.

ACHIEVING COMPETENCE

How are these skills to be learned? They will certainly not be learned in the classroom or the library. Project 2000 regularly stresses that the planning of placements must entail new thinking and it is on this new thinking that the new nurses' competence for community based practice will stand or fall. Unfortunately, many nurse teachers and community nurses are still bound by old ideas of 'going out for a day with the district nurse' or 'visiting a day centre'. Community nurses may feel that the constant 'company' of a student slows down their 'real' work and inhibits their relationships with their patients; nurse teachers who have never practised outside acute hospital settings may find it difficult to imagine what community based practice 'is like'. In the best Project 2000 programmes, however, experience is showing that such fears and limitations are unnecessary.

For example, acquiring skills in reflection and learning about participant and non-participant observation in other parts of their course enables students to gain new insights into their own and other people's behaviour in ordinary social settings — thinking about food choices in a supermarket, or smoking behaviour in a pub; watching children in a playground or elderly people on a bus; sitting in a general practitioner's surgery waiting room or a hospital outpatient department (a study of normal anxiety); watching men working on a building site (count the environmental hazards); attending a funeral. The possibilities are infinite and the right kind of preparation and follow-up can make them rich learning experiences.

With a little support, students are well able to negotiate their own 'placements' as volunteers in a variety of community groups and informal care agencies, developing their organisational and negotiating skills in the process; they can conduct surveys of health behaviour, morbidity, or health service usage among their friends and peers without infringing research ethics; they can gain some small insight into the experience of disability by trying to get around town in a wheelchair; they can use published data to begin to learn about community assessment and to develop community profiles.

Only after this should students progress to more privileged settings such as community based health and social service facilities to which access needs to be negotiated and patient and client interests protected by a responsible health professional. These facilities might include day nurseries, schools, day care centres, group homes, workplaces (often best seen through the eyes of an occupational health nurse), clinics of all kinds, and GP surgeries. Accompanying nurses into people's homes may be a relatively small and relatively later part of the programme and may be more meaningful if it is linked with learning about nursing practice related to particular groups such as children, elderly people, people with mental health problems and people suffering from chronic illness.

The student's supernumerary status provides much more freedom to structure learning time than in the past and it is important that they take responsibility for organising it. They need time to prepare for and reflect on their practice. 'Clinical learning' is not necessarily synonymous with 'being on the ward'. The expression of EC and National Board requirements as numbers of hours is counter-productive if it is interpreted rigidly.

There are excellent examples for new courses to follow. In several places students are asked to develop a profile of a defined community; the information to be collected (which may require library research, empirical data, observational visits and discussions with health professionals and others in a wide range of settings) includes the population profile, environmental influences on health, description of local services, people's use and perceptions of 'health services', facilities for disabled people, etc. This kind of exercise has been part of health visitor education for many years. In some places, students are introduced at an early stage in their programme to a family whose health and health care experiences they monitor over a long period. They can follow individual patients from community to hospital and hospital to community; attaching the student to the patient may provide much more opportunity for learning than attachment to a nurse or a ward or a particular clinical setting.

These approaches are a radical departure from traditional practices and need to be recognised as such. Teachers, clinical staff (in both hospital and community) and students themselves need to break away from old stereotypes and may need considerable help to do so. Nurse teachers who have no experience of community nursing will need specific re-orientation programmes (including placements in community clinical settings) (WHO 1991).

Planned visits and exchanges between hospital and community nurses who are working with students as perceptors are an equally important investment and changing public as well as professional stereotypes of nursing and of the student nurse requires a major public relations effort.

The Royal College of Nursing's Task Force on Community Nursing took as its starting point the view expressed in the English *Strategy for Nursing* document that:

> 'If the role of the nurse is first and foremost to respond to human needs, and in today's world these needs are continually and rapidly changing, then the nursing profession must change with them.' (Department of Health 1989)

Change is rarely easy. As Machiavelli wrote:

> 'There is nothing more difficult, more perilous to conduct or more uncertain in its success than to take the lead in a new order of things, because the innovator has for enemies all those who have done well under the old system and lukewarm defenders in those who *may* do well under the new.' (Machiavelli 1970)

But nursing has to change, and Project 2000 now provides an opportunity for nurses to move in the right direction. Perhaps Florence Nightingale was right even about the timing when with the most amazing prescience she wrote:

> 'I look to the abolition of all hospitals and workhouse infirmaries — but no use to talk about the year 2000 . . . !'

REFERENCES

Altschul A (1989) One or Many? Keynote address to the CNAA Training Conference 1989. *Community Psychiatric Nursing Journal*, **9**, 6, 14–18.

Baly M (1991) *As Miss Nightingale Said*. London: Scutari Press.

Department of Health (1989) Strategy for Nursing. London: HMSO.

Machiavelli N (1970) *The Prince*. London: Penguin.

Mahler H (1987) A Powerhouse for Change. *Senior Nurse*, **6**, 3, 23.

Nursing Times (Editorial) (1993) The wrong way to help. *Nursing Times*, **89**, 2, 3.

UKCC (1986) *Project 2000: A New Preparation for Practice*. London: UKCC.

WHO (1974) *Community Health Nursing: Report of an Expert Committee*. WHO Technical Report Series no. 558. Geneva: WHO.

WHO (1978)*Primary Health Care*. (Health For All Series no 1). Geneva: WHO.

WHO (1982) *Nursing in Support of the Goal of Health for All by the Year 2000*. HMD/NUR/82.2. Geneva: WHO.

WHO (1985) *Targets for Health For All* (European Health For All series no. 1). Copenhagen: WHO.

WHO (1987) *People's Needs for Nursing Care: a European Study*. Copenhagen: WHO.

WHO (1989) *European Conference on Nursing*. Copenhagen: WHO.

WHO (1991a) *Mission and Functions of the Nurse. Health For All*. Nursing Series no. 2. Copenhagen: WHO.

WHO (1991b) *Reviewing and Reorienting the Basic Nursing Curriculum*. Health for All Nursing Series no. 5. Copenhagen: WHO.

FURTHER READING

DHSS (1986) *Neigbourhood Nursing: A Focus for Care* (report of the Review of Community Nursing in England). London: HMSO.

Mahler H (1987) A powerhouse for change. *Senior Nurse,* **6**, 3, 23.

McMurray A (1990) *Community Health Nursing: Primary Health Care in Practice.* Edinburgh: Churchill Livingstone.

O'Neill P (1982) *Health Crisis 2000.* London: Heinemann.

WHO Regional Office for Europe. *Health for All Nursing Series.*
  No. 1 Health For All: the nursing mandate.
  No. 2 Mission and Functions of the Nurse.
  No. 3 The Nursing in Action Project.
  No. 4 Reviewing and Re-orienting the Basic Nursing Curriculum.

WHO (1989) *European Conference on Nursing* (includes Vienna Declaration on Nursing in Support of the European Targets for Health For All). Copenhagen: WHO.

CHAPTER 9

The Changing Face of Nursing — 2000 and Beyond

Jean Thomas and Brian Dolan

'The future is called "perhaps", which is the only possible thing to call the future. And the important thing is not to let it scare you'
(Tennessee Williams)

INTRODUCTION

Initiating and responding to change is a major requirement of today's workforce. While change itself is not new, what has become increasingly evident throughout the 1990's is the rate at which change takes place.

Nursing has seen a considerable number of developments in the past 10 years. Some, like the RCN Standards of Care Dynamic Standard Setting System (DySSSy) Project (RCN 1990) and the Nurse Prescribing Act (1992) have been initiated by the Royal College of Nursing, others in recognised nursing research centres such as Chelsea College, Oxford Institute of Nursing and The Royal Marsden Academic Research Unit. Centres of excellence have been established by the inspiration and commitment of nursing leaders committed to the individualisation and continuity of care and the development of nursing. Such centres have been aptly termed Nursing Development Units, the most notable examples being located at Oxford and Tameside (Pearson 1988).

Looking to the future, nursing faces an enormous, yet exciting challenge ahead in equipping today's nurse to function in tomorrow's world. The nurse will need to function within:

— a profession which is becoming more innovative,
— a less traditional/predictable working environment,
— a more commercial and competitive working environment,
— a world where high technological satellite centres will replace traditional hospital settings,
— a society where those who are alone, vulnerable or infirm will be re-directed to centres of convalescence of a hotel nature rather than prolong their stay in hospital,

A PROFESSION WHICH IS BECOMING MORE INNOVATIVE

Knowledge is the basis upon which clinical judgement is made (Benner 1984). No longer can practitioners rely on knowledge gained during initial nurse training as the life span of previously learned knowledge becomes shorter. This can be a painful experience for some practitioners who discover that a life-long ideology has been rendered invalid as a result of scientific testing (Duberly cited in Johns 1991). It is not uncommon to witness a reactive response to this discovery (Marris 1984).

Nonetheless, practitioners are expected by the nature of their professional Code of Conduct (UKCC, 1992) to

'maintain and improve your professional knowledge and competence'.

Such opportunities are not always freely available within the public or private sectors owing to the pressure of financial restraints. With nurses' pay consuming a 3 in 100 proportion of total public expenditure, this is not entirely surprising (Buchan and Ball 1991).

There remains a gap between the theory and practice of nursing (Millar 1985) despite substantial investment. The results of nursing research are not yet fully implemented in everyday practice. For instance, the research findings to support the aetiology and prophylaxis of decubitus ulcers is all too rarely utilised. Such indifference to the outcome of clinical research is not seen so frequently in medical practice. If, for example, a medical practitioner prescribed a Kaolin poultice for the treatment of a chest infection rather than antibiotics, such action could have serious medico-legal consequences.

Changes in nurse education such as Project 2000 will undoubtedly help bridge the gap between innovation and application but there still remains a vacuum and a need to interpret and communicate results from centres for innovation and research to the nurse at the bedside. One example of this has been by the Standards of Care DySSSy project (RCN 1990), which enables practitioners to evaluate and re-evaluate the standards of care they deliver.

Nurse managers, teachers and practitioners will continue to be catalysts for change as interpreters/communicators of nursing developments. Specialist nursing associations are an excellent medium for this kind of communication and such groups should be strengthened and supported in every way as they serve to promote specialism within nursing. It is these clinical specialist roles that are usually associated with an appropriate, usually medically defined, field of practice, such as diabetes care or stoma therapy. Other specialist roles have also emerged to meet client needs as well as an expansion of nursing knowledge, such as bereavement counsellors, palliative care nurses and continence promotion advisers (Wright 1992).

Such knowledge equips practitioners with the confidence to challenge traditional or unsafe practice. Generalists are ill equipped and may over-rely on medical direction. If nursing is to remain autonomous, then we need to support the concept of specialism while maintaining a spirit of commonality.

Nurses when they work together can make change happen. Witness, for instance, Project 2000, or clinical grading. A successful outcome from persistent lobbying has resulted in the Access to Health Records Act (1991) and the adoption of the 'named nurse' concept in the Patient's Charter (1992). Never before has nursing been afforded such opportunities and it is essential that such achievements become a reality in everyday practice.

Those faced with the challenge of implementation may be confronted with many obstacles from managers and colleagues. Some nurses undertaking this role are apprehensive when faced with more clearly defined levels of accountability (Manthey 1980). Such apprehension is inevitable as practitioners become autonomous and responsible for their own practice.

As it develops, nursing practice will become less prescriptive as practitioners grow in confidence and expertise. This will occasionally cause conflict with doctors and other professionals who are accustomed to nurses working in a traditional subordinate role (Buckenham and McGrath 1983; Luty 1992). In the longer term, true teamwork can only develop if nurses are able to function as full and equal team members (Reid and Price 1992).

A LESS TRADITIONAL/PREDICTABLE WORKING ENVIRONMENT

For the hospital nurse, future organisation of care is more likely to be arranged as client case load rather than holding responsibility for an environment of care, such as a ward or defined clinical area. This could have the positive effect of relieving practitioners of their 'hotelier' responsibilities, enabling them to deliver care uninterrupted, much like their community colleagues. Any remaining responsibility for hotel services and supplies will become the province of hotel service staff as cost containment seeks to maximise the professional skills of nurses.

Greater emphasis upon continuity of care and the named nurse/midwife concept may well lead to increasing use of the Domino (DOMiciliary IN-Out) system used extensively in midwifery, which places the emphasis of the pregnancy in the community. It also individualises and humanises care argues Rundell (1992) because:

> 'You cannot truly appreciate the effect that the interpersonal relationship has on care until you have been on the receiving end.' (p. 24)

Traditional methods of nurse training have up until now restricted the hospital nurse from practising in the community. Project 2000 at last lays the foundation for the development of a more generic practitioner who will be enskilled to practise in both institutional and non-institutional settings (UKCC 1986). Shifting certain types of acute and terminal care through 'hospital at home' schemes will further blur the distinctions between medical and nursing practitioners (Taylor 1989) and hospital and community settings.

In mental health and learning disabilities care, the client profile will change dramatically as the impact of genetic screening and counselling is felt. As scientists seek to identify all 100 000 human genes by the year 2005, it not only promises to transform our understanding of what makes us biologically, but tantalises us with the prospect of altering, for better or worse, what we may become (Cornwell 1992). If it is possible to identify the genetic predisposition for schizophrenia or Down's syndrome, what social, scientific and ethical implications will we see? One effect is, right or wrong, that there will almost certainly be fewer babies with learning disabilities born.

The introduction of multi-speciality day case units and the possibility of Graduated Patient Care will accentuate the need for peripatetic practice (Thomas 1992 unpublished). Specialist nursing skills must be nurtured for the benefit of clients, they cannot be allowed to waste by merely changing the environment of care with the added risk of nurses practising outside their field of competence. The nurse, where appropriate, must be able to follow the client and be sufficiently skilled and adaptable to care in any environment, be it the ward, day case unit or community.

A MORE COMMERCIAL AND COMPETITIVE WORKING ENVIRONMENT

Nurses who practise within the new internal market of the NHS are being subject to the same pressures as those employed within the commercial world of the private sector. The workforce size has remained almost static, with growth averaging only 0.2 per cent a year between 1983 and 1987. However, over the same period, the total workload, as measured by the number of in-patient and day cases, has increased by more than 4 per cent a year (HM Treasury cited in Beardshaw 1992).

The probability of performance related pay begs the question of what are and who will decide upon the performance criteria. When conflict exists between return on investment and quality of care, how often are the co-operation and loyalties sought by the manager from the nursing staff bought in the form of a pay rise? A frequent scenario experienced by those employed in the independent sector is one of the manager receiving a performance related increase of 35 per cent for exceeding revenue forecasts. The nurse manager may be rewarded to the tune of 10–15 per cent and the nurse at the bedside is awarded a 2–6 per cent annual increase.

For this, the clinical practitioner may have cared for three patients in each bed per day; one prior to discharge, one day case and one evening admission for surgery the following day. Such care is delivered in an environment where lack of clinical error or omission may be due more to luck than judgement. Generally this pay award is in the region of £200 per annum above that offered to health service nurses whose hospital or community units have not (yet) 'opted out' of NHS control. This constitutes an increase of £13 a week with less holiday entitlement and very little in the form of staff development, apart from the compulsory training in marketing skills to promote the (independent sector) hospital.

In a commercial world, employers will generally pay what they can 'get away with'. Where such bargaining takes place, the deal is secured by the party able to demonstrate better negotiating skills. Historically, this has been the domain of the unions who negotiate on behalf of their members. Such skills are not yet part of a nurse's initial training programme nor are their caring skills seen as compatible with having to succeed in a competitive world. As has been demonstrated in the independent sector, where health service unions do not have negotiating rights, nurses become victims until they learn to appreciate their value in the market place and are assisted in the art of promoting and negotiating for themselves.

While much discussion has taken place on the subject of empowering patients (Wright 1986; Dolan 1991; Crane 1991), there is an assumption that nurses are sufficiently empowered to protect themselves. Where national agreements are replaced by local pay bargaining, it is essential that nurses learn to articulate their professional value and negotiate their rightful recognition. The increased input on assertiveness and interpersonal skills in Project 2000 curricula will give nurses much of the self-confidence they require to speak up for themselves as well as their clients and patients.

HIGH TECHNOLOGY SATELLITE CENTRES

The rising cost of capital equipment due to technological advancement will result in such technology being centred in a few regionally selected areas. Traditional in-patient care delivery will become the exception. The main changes will arise from improvements in less invasive surgical technologies, laser, catheters, improved imaging and diagnostic techniques.

The services of these centres may be purchased nationally. They will be able to provide diagnostic and non-invasive intervention on an outpatient or day case basis. Decreasing use of general anaesthesia as a result of more sophisticaed sedatives and better local anaesthesia will lessen recovery time.

Such advancement cannot take place without further changes in the workplace. Technological centres with non-invasive intervention will replace the traditional operating theatre. Many procedures previously carried out by surgeons will become the domain of ambulatory physicians and radiologists. Technological advancement in the management of pain will be carried out by anaesthetists/ pain physicians in these new centres. The changes in medical practice will result in the transfer of medical power away from the clinicians to the technological specialists from the laboratory and radiology departments (Jolly 1990).

The consequences for nursing may be found in combining the skills of theatre, x-ray, out-patient and ward nurses, all of whom will have to work in these new centres alongside technicians and radiographers. The introduction of the more generic health care assistant will serve to complicate further the lines of accountability and responsibility.

Those nurses more accustomed to caring for patients who are anaesthetised will need to increase their awareness of the behavioural sciences. The increasing technological sophistication of acute care, coupled with the countervailing pressures to devise more humane and individually-centred approaches to health problems of all types, will demand new responses and skills from health care workers (Beardshaw and Robinson 1991).

The importance of continuity of care cannot be overstressed, particularly where there is increasing patient turnover (Beardshaw 1991). Much like the USA, this environment lends itself to the peripatetic perioperative nurse, who becomes the 'named nurse'; the one who makes contact with the client prior to the intervention, accompanies the client throughout the intervention and maintains contact after discharge. The custom of clients being admitted to a ward by a ward nurse and then passed on to a theatre nurse or technician is both fragmented and expensive. The perioperative nurse of the future can expect to work in 'partnership' with clients. The term implying the relationship between carer and client is essentially an equal one (Savage 1987).

This new role also offers opportunities for theatre nurses whose current role is under threat amidst cost containment exercises. While cost is easier to measure than quality (Buchan 1990), Project 2000 nurses will have useful skills of a health educative, rather than disease orientated role in meeting the needs of a less compliant, more informed and empowered client group.

HOTEL-LIKE CENTRES OF CONVALESCENCE

The concept of a society where those who are alone, vulnerable or infirm will be directed to hotel-like centres of convalescence originated in the USA (Bradley-Davis and Groneman 1987). It was initiated by clients themselves because of the rising costs of hospitalisation and ambulatory transport to return home. In the UK this scheme has been considered for those 30–40 per cent of hospital in-patients who remain in acute hospital beds owing to social circumstances (RCN 1992).

The cost of such hospitalisation far exceeds that of hotel accommodation and it is debatable whether optimum recovery can take place in such an acute setting. Hospitalisation for social reasons also serves to accentuate the loneliness of this group and promotes feelings of guilt when the individual knows he or she is blocking a bed for someone else.

For nurses the decision to discharge a patient to a hotel-like centre of convalescence will be easier than discharging home someone who lives alone. One effect of this change, however, will be to increase the workload of community nurses as some patients will require wound dressings and assessment prior to returning home.

A more efficient use of the remaining acute beds could offer a better service for those awaiting admission and a reduction in the number seeking private health care. At the same time, the addition of 30–40 per cent more acutely ill, rather than convalescent patients, requires additional resources for staffing. This should involve a collaborative review of numbers and skill mix to reflect the changes to both the nursing workload and provision of care (Audit Commission 1992). The redirection of patients from hospital to hotel may in some instances benefit the client, but it is not a cheaper option for managers.

For those caring for people with learning disabilities or mental health problems, nurses will increasingly work as independent practitioners to whom patients and clients can have direct access (Hancock 1990). They will provide the skilled, but invisible support which will enable many hundreds of thousands of people to remain in their own or group homes, despite chronic conditions or illness, thus providing an enhanced quality of life.

SUMMARY

As we leave the 20th Century the emphasis will continue to move from hospital to community. Nurses will play a more pro-active role in the maintenance of health and in providing primary, secondary and tertiary health education. Nurses of the 21st Century will be actively involved in directing change and be adaptable in a changing world without fear of that change.

For the Project 2000 nurse it is a time not to fear, but to celebrate the future and to make the most of the opportunities available to nurses and nursing. At times it may be challenging, but in the words of Barbara Vaughan (1989):

'Without risk, there would be no growth.'

REFERENCES

Access to Health Records Act (1991) London: HMSO.

Audit Commission (1992) *The Virtue of Patients: Making Best Use of Ward Nursing Resources*. London: HMSO.

Beardshaw V (1992) Prospects for Nursing. In *In the Best of Health?: The status and future of health care in the UK* (eds E Beck, S Lonsdale, S Newman and D Patterson) London: Chapman & Hall.

Beardshaw V and Robinson K (1991) *New for Old?: Prospects for Nursing*. London: King's Fund Institute.

Benner P (1984) *From Novice to Expert: Excellence and Power in Clinical Nursing Practice*. Menlo Park: Addison-Wesley.

Bradley-Davis M L and Groneman S (1987) The hotel alternative program: a new trend for cost-containment. *ANNA Journal*, **14**, 1, 22–4.

Buchan J (1990) The Shape of the Future. *Nursing Times*, **86**, 25, 19.

Buchan J and Ball J (1991) *Caring Costs*. IMS Report No 208. Brighton: Institute of Manpower Services.

Buckenham J and McGrath G (1983) *The Social Reality of Nursing*. Sydney: Adis.

Cornwell J (1992) Gene Spleen. *Sunday Times Magazine*, July 26, 16–21.

Crane S (1991) Implications of the critical paradigm. In *Towards a Discipline of Nursing* (eds G Gray and R Pratt). Melbourne: Churchill Livingstone.

Department of Health (1992) *The Patients' Charter*. London: HMSO.

Dolan B (1991) Power to the Project? *Nursing Standard*, **5**, 28, 47.

Hancock C (1990) *21st Century Nurse: Home Thoughts From Abroad*. 1990 Kathleen Raven Lecture. London: RCN.

Johns C (1991) Introducing and Managing Change — The Move to Primary Nursing. In *Primary Nursing in Perspective* (eds S Ersser and E Tutton) London: Scutari Press.

Jolly M (1990) Medicine 2000 — Forecasting the Future of Health Care, Conference Paper, BUPA Symposium (unpublished).

Luty J (1992) A Primary Complaint. *Nursing Times* (Letters), **88**, 26, 14.
Manthey M (1980) *The Practice of Primary Nursing*. Boston: Blackwell Scientific.
Marris P (1984) *Loss and Change*. London: Routledge and Kegan Paul.
Millar A (1985) The relationship between nursing theory and nursing practice. *Journal of Advanced Nursing*, **10**, 5, 417–24.
Nurse Prescribing Act (1992) London: HMSO.
Pearson A (1988) *Primary Nursing: Nursing in the Burford and Oxford Nursing Development Units*, London: Croom Helm.
Reid B and Price J (1992) Is Primary Nursing Keeping The Doctors Happy? *Nursing Times* (Letters), **88**, 30, 15.
Royal College of Nursing (1990) *Standards of Care Project. Quality Patient Care: The Dynamic Standard Setting System*. London: Scutari Press.
Royal College of Nursing (1992) *Hospital Hotels*. RCN Annual Congress (Matter for Discussion). London: RCN.
Rundell S (1992) The Domino Effect. *Nursing Times*, **88**, 29, 24.
Savage J (1987) *Nurses, Gender and Sexuality*. London: Heinemann.
Taylor D. (1989) *Hospital at Home: The coming revolution*. London: King's Fund Centre.
United Kingdom Central Council for Nursing, Midwifery and Health Visiting (1986) *Project 2000: A New Preparation for Practice*. London: UKCC.
United Kingdom Central Council for Nursing, Midwifery and Health Visiting (1992) *Code of Professional Conduct* (Third Edition). London: UKCC.
Vaughan B (1989) Accountability and Autonomy. *Nursing Times*, **85**, 3, 54–55.
Wright S (1986) *Building and Using a Model of Nursing*. London: Edward Arnold.
Wright S (1992) Advances in clinical practice. *British Journal of Nursing*, **1**, 4, 192–4.

Public Statements on Nurse Education

1. *The Lancet Commission (1932)*
   Proposed:
   — Pre-nursing courses
   — Ward sisters freed from other duties for teaching
   — Endowment funding for trainees

2. *Inter-departmental Committee on Nursing Services (Athlone Report) (1938)*
   Proposed:
   — A two-part preliminary and a final examination
   — The first part preliminary taken as a pre-nursing course

3. *The Nursing Reconstruction Committee (Horder Report) (1941–1949)*
   Proposed:
   — Fewer/larger training schools
   — Entry by school certificate or alternative entrance test
   — Training broader: preventive and social medicine included
   — A revitalised GNC with an inspectorate
   — A generic training with post-basic courses

4. *Working Party on the Recruitment and Training of Nurses (Wood Report) (1947)*
   Majority Report
   Proposed:
   — Regional training boards
   — Student status

— 18 months' generic course followed
by 6 months' specialist training

Minority Report (Cohen Report) (1948)
— Dissented on grounds that until
future demands of new NHS are
ascertained the role (and thus the
training) of nurses was in question

5. *Report of the Working Party on Midwives (Stocks Report) (1949)*
   Proposed:
   — Student midwives should have
   student status linked to case
   assignment
   — Single integrated midwifery training
   (as opposed to Part 1 and Part 2
   training)
   — That there is no inherent reason
   why midwife students should be
   SRN unless specialist training for
   SRN's to train as midwives is
   developed
   — Specialist training for midwifery
   following a general course should
   be of one year's duration (Wood
   Report had proposed six months)
   — Schools of midwifery should be
   separate from schools of nursing
   and the hospital system

6. *Committee on Higher Education (Robbins Report) (1963)*
   Proposed:
   — Nursing outwith the concerns of
   higher education

7. *A Reform of Nurse Education (Platt Report) (1964)*
   Proposed:
   — Regional councils for nurse
   education
   — Fewer schools
   — Nurse education independent from
   NHS and exchequer funded
   — Student status and educational
   grants
   — 5 'O' level entry or equivalent
   — Two-year broader training with
   one-year supervised practice
   — Links with higher education
   — More degree courses

8. *Committee on Nursing (Briggs Report) (1972)*
   Proposed: — Larger 'colleges'
   — Selection by aptitude and intelligence, not 'O' levels alone
   — Modular training
   — 18 month 'certificate in nursing practice' course (a generic course), followed by 18 month specialist registration courses

9. *Royal Commission on the National Health Service (Merrison Report) (1979)*
   Proposed: — Support for Briggs
   — More nurse teachers
   — Development of research capacity

10. *Committee of Enquiry into Mental Handicap Nursing and Care (Jay Report) (1979)*
    Proposed: — Nurses not adequately prepared for this field
    — Transfer of care to social services

11. *The Preparation and Education of Teachers of Nursing (Chapman Report) (1983)*
    Proposed: — One grade of nurse teacher
    — Teaching courses to have a 'professional' as well as 'educational' component
    — Increase in graduate teachers
    — In each college, a teacher trained in:
      1. Advanced education administration
      2. Research methodology
    — Development of teaching role of ward managers

12. *GNCs/CCETSW — Co-operation in Training — Parts I and II (1982/83)*
    Proposed: — Co-operation in training between mental handicap nursing and social work
    — Joint RNMH/CCS course at qualifying level
    — Co-operation and sharing at post-qualifying level

13. *The Education of Nurses: A New Dispensation — Commission on Nurse Education (Judge Report) (1985)*

    Proposed:
- Nurse education out of NHS into higher education
- Three-year diploma course, for a single grade of nurse
- Five 'specialties, with specialism in final year after two "generic" years of study'
- 5 'O' level entry, student status and student bursaries rather than salaries

14. *Project 2000 — UKCC (1986)*

    Proposed:
- One *new* level of nurse
- Common foundation programme up to two years
- 'Branching' programmes for each major division of nursing leading to registration (but on experimental basis for midwifery, for which there is a status quo situation)
- New set of competencies
- Larger training institutions
- Links with higher education
- Student status and bursaries

UKCC A New Preparation for Practice — 1986 Summary of Project 2000 Recommendations

1. There should be a new registered nurse competent to assess the need for care, provide care, monitor and evaluate and to do this in institutional and non-institutional settings.
2. Preparation for registration should normally be completed within three years.
3. All preparation for registration should begin with a common foundation programme followed by branch programmes.
4. The common foundation programme should be a substantial part of preparation, lasting up to two years.
5. Branch programmes should be available, in mental illness, mental handicap, nursing adults and nursing children, with experimentation in a branch for midwifery.
6. In the case of midwifery, there should also be an 18 months' post-registration preparation.
7. There should be a new, single list of competencies applicable to all registered practitioners at the level of registration and set out in Training Rules.
8. All future practitioners should register with Council. The area of practice should be indicated on the register.
9. Midwives should debate the new registered practitioner outcomes in the light of their special needs.
10. There should be a coherent, comprehensive, cost-effective framework of education beyond registrations.
11. There should be specialist practitioners, some of whom will also be team leaders, in all areas of practice in hospital and community settings. The requisite specialist qualifications will be recordable on Council's register.

12. Health visiting, occupational health visiting and school nursing should be specialist qualifications on health promotion which are recordable on Council's register.
13. District nursing, community psychiatric nursing and community mental handicap nursing should be specialist qualifications which are recordable on Council's register.
14. Students should be supernumerary to NHS staffing establishment throughout the whole period of preparation.
15. There should be a new helper grade, directly supervised and monitored by a registered practitioner.
16. Students should receive training grants which are primarily NHS-controlled. These grants should be administered via National Boards and should derive from a separately identified education budget.
17. The position of teaching staff should be improved with a view to enhancing performance and allowing teachers opportunities for further training and for full participation in wider educational activities.
18. The full range of options to achieve the appropriate concentrations of educational resources should be considered, including re-establishments, partnerships, consortia etc.
19. Educational costs should be clearly identified and heads of educational institutions should be given responsibility for management of a more comprehensive and clearly delineated education budget.
20. Practitioners should have formal preparation for teaching roles in practice settings.
21. Moves should be made to establish teaching qualifications at degree level for teachers of nursing, midwifery and health visiting.
22. Joint professional and academic validation should be pursued from the very outset of change, in order to achieve academic recognition for professional qualifications.
23. Programmes of training for entry to the EN parts of the register should cease as soon as practicable.
24. The enhancement of opportunities for ENs to enter RGN, RMN, RNMH, and RSCN parts of the register should be given priority.
25. Urgent consideration should be given to creating a new organisation structure to implement the proposals of Project 2000.

Vienna Declaration on Nursing in Support of the European Targets for Health For All

I

Health, which is a state of complete physical, mental and social wellbeing and not merely the absence of disease or infirmity, is a fundamental human right. The attainment of the highest possible level of health is a most important social goal, whose realisation requires the action of many professions.

II

The persisting inequalities in people's health status, both between and within countries of the WHO Europe Region, are politically, socially, economically and professionally unacceptable and therefore of common concern to all nurses.

III

Having provided nurses from the 32 countries in the Region with their first opportunity to re-examine their role, education and practice, the Conference reaffirms the status of nursing as a force that can make a major contribution to achieving the 38 targets adopted by the member states at the thirty-fourth session of the WHO Regional Committee for Europe in 1984.

IV

The participants pledge to bring the new role of the nurse in the era of health for all to the attention of ministries of health, the organisations and trade unions of all health professions, regulatory bodies and other groups throughout the Region. Nurses should develop their new role by: acting as partners in decision-making on the planning and management of local, regional and national health services, playing a greater role in empowering individuals, families and communities to become more self-reliant and to take charge of their health development, and providing clear and valid information on the favourable and adverse consequences of various types of behaviour, and on the merits and costs of different options for care.

V

New attitudes and values need to be fostered among all health professionals, health care consumers and related groups. These should be consistent with the directives and principles of health for all and primary health care. Nursing education must provide a sound foundation for nursing practice, especially work in the community, and nurses must take account of the social aspects of health needs and have a broader understanding of health development. Policies should be adopted and activities identified to enable nurses to practise with sufficient autonomy to carry out their role in primary health care.

VI

Research to improve practice along these lines should be encouraged through the creation of research policies and financial support. Such research should use human resources efficiently, and ensure the evaluation and use of its results. Nurses should also be involved in the research process.

Index

academic credibility   23, 60, 90
academic recognition   7
Access to Health Records Act
    1991   123
accountability   127
administration   32
advocacy   66
Alma Ata Declaration   112
altruism   68
androgogy   59
apprenticeship   4
assertiveness   52, 67
Association of Nursing Students   5
Athlone Report   131
awareness   64

Bottomley, Virginia   26
Briggs Report   21, 32, 33–4, 98–9,
    133
bullying   18, 20–1

Caines, Eric   25
career paths   13–14
  and marriage   82
  men's   81
caring   68, 78
change, psychology of   35–6
Chapman Report   133
Clarke, Kenneth   8, 23, 26
clinical experience   96–7
clinical grading   12, 123
clinical practice   89–102
clinical supervision   97

Cohen, John   20
Cohen Report   132
COHSE   8, 22, 84
Common Foundation Programme
    6, 7, 52, 64, 71–2
communication   52, 115
community care   6
Community Education and Practice
    101
community nursing   39, 100–1, 107
community practice   114–15
compassion   78
competence   115
complementary therapy   80
confidentiality   44
conformity   98
control, personal   41, 63
convalescence   128
conversion courses   99
culture, nursing   53

day care units   125
demographic change   6, 23, 24–5
dependency   68
disempowerment   64, 65
Domino system   124
DySSSy   121, 123

education, pre-registration   59, 72,
    91
elitism   90
empathy   64
empowerment   45, 57, 60–6, 126

ENB Framework for Continuing
  Education   100
enrolled nurse   7, 23, 98–9
  black   92
equal opportunities   69–70
ethnicity   69–70, 92
European Conference on Nursing
  112

financial accountability   25

gender   68, 69, 75–87
General Nursing Council (GNC)
  4, 5, 19
generic health care   127
generic practitioner   124
genetic screening/counselling   124
goals   64
graduate nurses   11–13
graduate teachers   48
graduated patient care   125
Griffiths Report   32

health care   109
health care assistants   35, 98
  black   70
health promotion   110
high-tech centres   126–7
high-tech nursing   68, 79
high-touch nursing   79
higher education   34, 48, 56, 94–8
holistic care   37
homosexuality   78
Horder Report   3, 20, 131
hospital at home scheme   124
hospitalisation   128
hotel-like centres   27, 125

ICN   112
inequality   91–2
information   65
intellectualism   90–1

Jay Report   133
Judge Report   6–7, 21, 22, 134

Lancet Commission   131
language   70–1
learning disabilities   124–5
learning, student-centred   58–60
lifeskills   65
locus of control   62, 63

Mahler, Halfdan   113
management   32
  male-dominated   80–1
marginalisation   70
marriage   84
masculinity   79
matrons   18
mature students   69, 93–4
mental health care   124, 128
mentors   84
Merrison Report   133
Mohammed, Safder   92
morale   65
Moore, John   8, 23

named nurse   123, 124, 127
NHS Act 1990   85
NHS reform   25
Nightingale School   18
NUPE   84
nurse career progress   11, 13
nurse–doctor relationship   66–7
nurse education reform   6, 7, 22,
  23, 54
nurse, graduate   11–12
nurse, male   68, 69, 75
nurse management   81
nurse–patient relationship   62
nurse, perioperative   127
Nurse Prescribing Act 1992   121
nurse teachers   95–6
nurse, theatre   127
nurse training   4, 17, 18
nurse, undergraduate   9–10
  isolation of   95
Nursing Development Units   80,
  121
nursing, general   71
nursing, hands-on   18
nursing, image of   42

nursing, men's role 76
nursing, research-based 18, 34
nursing theory 34
nursing values 97

observation 116

passivity 68
patient-centred care 61–2
patriarchy 67, 79
pay bargaining 126
pay, performance-related 125
Pay Review Body 9
perioperative nurse 127
placements 97, 116
  ward-based 38
Platt Report 5, 21, 132
powerlessness 62
practice, research-based 18
PREPP 100
primary health care 80, 109, 110
Project 2000 134
  funding 26
  government approval 8
  reception 9
  resistance to 38–41
  summary 135–6
psychology 52

racism 69–70, 92–3
reflection 116
registered nurse 98
registration, simple 98
research 27, 52
  ethics 116
responsibility 127
Robbins Report 132
Royal College of Nursing (RCN)
  4, 6, 84, 117

Salmon Report 80–1
scientism 60
self-empowerment 63–6
self-perpetuation 17

sexism 70, 81
sexuality 79
simple registration 98
skills 115
  academic 37, 40–1
  behavioural 65, 116
  interpersonal 64
  negotiating 116, 126
  practical 42
  reflection 116
social change 89
social conditioning 54
social groups
  dominant 69
  subordinate 68
social representation 32–4
specialisation 49
specialist practitioners 114,
  123
staff support groups 65
staffing levels 23–24
status 32
  apprenticeship 21
  graduate 12, 48
  social 39
  student 19–20, 47–8
  supernumerary 4, 6, 33, 37, 39,
    42, 116–17
  women's 32
Stocks Report 132
stress 48
Student Bill of Rights 62
student-centred learning 58–60
Student Nurses Association 5
student parents 69
studentship 4
supernumerary status 4, 6, 33, 37,
  39, 42, 116–17
support workers 22, 23–4

teachers, graduate 47
teamwork 124
theatre nurse 127
theory–practice gap 50
tutor–student relationship 60

UKCC 7, 84

values 64
Vienna Declaration 137–8
virtues, female 78

whistleblowing 66
WHO 110, 111, 112
womanhood 68
Wood Report 4, 131